Jim Aylward,

I have enjoyed you years & I hope this book will serve as an introduction

Jim Reardon

Plastic Surgery for Men

Plastic Surgery for Men

THE COMPLETE ILLUSTRATED GUIDE

James J. Reardon, M.D.

AND

Judi McMahon

ILLUSTRATED BY HARRIET E. PHILLIPS

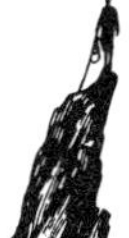

EVEREST HOUSE, PUBLISHERS, NEW YORK

Library of Congress Cataloging in Publication Data:
Reardon, James J
Plastic surgery for men.

Includes index.
1. Surgery, Plastic. 2. Men—Surgery.
I. McMahon, Judi, joint author. II. Title.
RD119.R43 1981 617'.95 80-29465
ISBN: 0-89696-069-2

Published simultaneously in Canada by
Beaverbooks, Don Mills, Ontario
Manufactured in the United States of America
Designed by Joyce Cameron Weston
First Edition RRD781

To my wife, Robin, for her patience
and understanding,
and to my parents for *their* help
and understanding during the
arduous years in the making of a
surgeon.

—James J. Reardon, M.D.

To Bill W. and his friends for making all of this possible, to Baba with love, and for my parents, Sylvia and Sam Kimmel

—Judi McMahon

ACKNOWLEDGMENTS

From James J. Reardon, M.D.:

"Many hands make light work," a quotation from a famous Chinese leader, expresses a great truth. Putting this book together required the skill and help of the following people, and I want them to know how much I appreciate their dedicated efforts:

Harriet E. Phillips for her patience and detailed illustrations and drawings; Vincent Maiello, my photographer, for the photographs he assembled; my office staff: Nicole Loening, Eileen Curlander, and my medical assistant, Michael Richheimer, and those patients whose stories and photographs have contributed so much to this book; office manager Vera Ricciardi, and my associate, Alvin Harris, M.D., whose assistance and advice have been invaluable to me.

And, to Judi McMahon, who came to me with this project, and whose perceptions and creative abilities have helped to make this book a reality, my very special appreciation and thanks for her enthusiasm, unswerving dependability, and special skills in creating a clear and readable guide out of the information I wanted to share with the public.

From Judi McMahon:

My own warm thank-you to you, Dr. James Reardon. Your love for your work, your good humor, and thorough professionalism were absolutely vital to the successful completion of this book. Busy as you were, you always found the time to check, recheck, and clarify the information within this guide. In the year and a half that we have worked together, I have never ceased to be impressed by the miracle of your art.

And to Jerry Gross, our editor, my deeply felt appreciation for his steadfast faith in this work, and for his excellent editing and creative guardianship throughout the endeavor. In the end, it was Jerry's patience and pragmatism that made this all possible.

Contents

Foreword

THERE HAVE BEEN many books in recent years on the subject of plastic surgery, but none directed toward the specific needs of a man. As much as 30 to 35 percent of my practice is now devoted to male plastic surgery. This represents a great increase over the last three to five years. Prior to that, as little as 10 percent of my practice was devoted to men.

My intention in this book is to explain everything a man might want to know about the art of cosmetic surgery. It is a challenging task to one more comfortable with a scalpel than a typewriter. Within these limitations, let me tell you who I am, and how and why I came to write this book.

It seems to me that the general public, and even some of my patients, aren't aware of the extensive and complex training that a plastic surgeon must receive. I have even had patients who of course knew that I was a plastic surgeon, but asked if I was "a doctor, too."

A plastic surgeon's education is rigorous. After attending medical school for four years, there is also one year of internship followed by four years of general surgery. It was only at this point that I was ready to spend two more years specializing, specifically, in plastic surgery.

By the time I started private practice, I was a relatively young thirty-one—and it had been fully seven years since I completed medical school. Throughout my training, I was able to observe many plastic surgeons perform and was influenced by the most brilliant of them.

The surgical training program at Kings County Hospital, in Brooklyn, New York, is one of the oldest in the country. Being a member of a complex municipal medical center gave me the opportunity to see many cases, ranging from facial lacerations to cancer disfigurations. There were not too many purely cosmetic cases at Kings County, but I was able to assist my professor when he worked with his private-patient case load at other hospitals. While as a novice I felt it was important to assist on all sorts of cases, I later realized that it is necessary to have seen many specific surgical procedures in each aspect of plastic surgery performed.

Since I first started in practice, attitudes toward plastic surgery have undergone a great change. No longer do I find that I have to be defensive about cosmetic surgery. I used to spend an extraordinary amount of time showing "before and after" pictures to prospective candidates, but no longer: my successful cases make my work self-evident. Most of those who consult with me know exactly what they want; there is little, if any, selling aspect at the initial consultation.

One recent patient came to see me because he wanted his jaw augmented. This young man had good dental occlusion and had undergone orthodontic work during his college years. He came to the office with his mother, who very much opposed the operation. I explained to her that times had changed; that attitudes had changed; that her son had the right to make up his own mind. He did. The operation was performed and he is so pleased with the outcome that he seems to have gained a new self-confidence. So much that even his mother commented on the positive change.

The satisfactions I receive from my work are indeed great. I see the results and I am aware of my patients' happiness. When the outcome is good, there is the joy of a job well done. Naturally, I make every effort to see that every operation turns out well. My only limitation is based on what I am working on—that is, the degree of reconstruction necessary and change that is possible.

Some of the more dramatic improvements are not necessarily cosmetic in nature. I recall a recent patient of mine who had carcinoma of the esophagus, which meant that the esophagus, along with his voice box, had to be totally removed. In the past, he would not have been able to speak or swallow, and would have had to be fed through a tube. But today there are procedures that allow for reconstruction of the swallowing mechanism of the alimentary tract. Although unable to talk, this patient can eat normally. I find such an operation particularly rewarding.

My work is filled with many such compensations. One of my patients had cancer of the nose. When the nose is totally reconstructed, he will be able to go back to work and feel as normal as possible.

There is also the more popular cosmetic rhinoplasty procedure, where a patient has his nose straightened or shortened and is relieved of an embarrassment or poor self-image he has felt for many years. That operation is also gratifying to the plastic surgeon.

Surgeons are human beings like anyone else. They appreciate praise. But, of course, they also know that not every procedure is an immediate success. A few years ago, a face-lift patient of mine developed a hematoma (swelling caused by bleeding beneath the skin) several hours after surgery. He was taken to the operating room at four o'clock in the morning, where I opened the stitches, removed the hematoma, and stitched him up again. That's a dramatic instance of things not going well. They happen, but they can be treated without affecting the final outcome. There are also those reconstructive cases where the result is a great improvement, but less than 100 percent satisfying. In most instances a subsequent procedure can correct these.

In this unique field, it might be worth noting that a plastic surgeon's results are there for everyone to see. One poor result can be disastrous for a surgeon's practice, particularly in a small community. Therefore it is imperative that a doctor not give his patients false promises and hopes, and that both agree on what can be accomplished satisfactorily—and that it is accomplished.

What kind of people are plastic surgeons? While you cannot go into a crowded room and point to a man with assurance and say that he is a plastic surgeon, there are probably some attributes that make us a breed apart. We are usually fastidious, neat, and meticulous. Generally we have a sense of beauty, balance, and proportion that carries through in our private lives. For instance, I raise orchids as a hobby. I also enjoy cooking. Other plastic surgeons paint or sculpt. And so on.

The life of a plastic surgeon may seem romantic and exciting, but there is also a great deal of dedication and discipline involved. I work six days a week, from six A.M. to eight P.M. On a typical day I may start out by going to the hospital and seeing patients on whom I operated the prior day. Meanwhile, between eight and nine A.M., that day's scheduled patients are being prepared for surgery. I meet and talk with them, as well as others who come for follow-up visits to my office. I begin operating at nine in the morning, and often keep going until one, two, or three in the afternoon. This means two or three cases have been done, depending on the complexity of each procedure. From three o'clock on I see new patients. I arrive home at about eight.

During most weeks I manage to find the time to teach residents at Kings County Hospital and at Methodist Hospital, both in Brooklyn, New York. At Kings County there are three residents a year in training for plastic surgery, and at Methodist one, who will also be board eligible in plastic surgery. It's not compulsory to teach, but I feel the obligation to pass on knowledge, just as other surgeons taught me when I was a resident.

There used to be stories about surgeons who liked to keep their techniques under wraps for fear that a "competitor" might learn special "tricks." Fortunately those days are gone. Today's surgeons are more than glad to pass on what they know to residents. In a teaching hospital, by the way, it is often a resident who is doing the actual cutting, under the direction of an attending surgeon. But remember that when a plastic surgery resident picks up a scalpel, he has already had at least three to four years' experience in general surgery. By the end of his two years of specialized training he will have done a considerable amount of plastic surgery.

In essence, this is how I became a surgeon, and also what my feelings are toward my patients and my practice. I truly enjoy what I do. And I hope that this guide will help you to understand cosmetic surgery and remove any fears you may have about it, as well as furnish you with all the specifics you need to help you decide whether you want to consider cosmetic surgery and discuss your problem with a plastic surgeon.

James J. Reardon, M.D.

New York, N.Y.
March, 1981

PART ONE

The Overview

ONE

The Male Candidate for Plastic Surgery

PLASTIC SURGERY has long recognized the human yearning for self-improvement. It was Gaspare Tagliacozzi, who is best known for his reconstructions of the mutilated face, who started way back in 1597. He said, "We restore, repair, and make whole parts which nature hath given, but which *fortune* hath taken away."

There have been times, though, when cosmetic improvement was not looked on with favor. The Victorian era viewed cosmetic surgery as both vain and sinful. Although physicians practiced cosmetic surgery as early as 1900, there is very little written about this period. The social prejudice against it continued through the first decades of this century, as physicians, reflecting the views of the culture, believed that the only valid reason for surgery was to save lives.

The early twentieth-century view of masculine attractiveness was a restrictive one. Men wore dark, conservative clothes, and hair styles that required a monthly visit to the barber. Apart from a wedding ring, a man's acceptable adornment was a stickpin, watch fob, or cufflinks. Most men had a stark, unimaginative, and utilitarian sameness about them. Along with this drab demeanor, men had to maintain the image of always being tough, rugged, cool, dominant, and distant. They were condemned to project a false image—one of bravado. There was no relief from the rigid facade they had to maintain.

It wasn't until the 1950s that attitudes began to change. Television—then a fast-growing, popular medium—projected a new message in bars and living rooms across the country. Men began to listen intently to those after-shave commercials featuring the middleweight champion raving about his newly smooth jawline. If rough and tough sports figures used and recommended a "beauty product," it must be masculine. For who could be more representative of virility, maleness, and even machismo than an athlete?

In the sixties, America produced not only the women's movement but also a new definition of the masculine value system that led to what was termed the "liberated" male. It was the age of encounter groups and letting go. Men started to free themselves of the stereotypes that limited them in their ability to show sensitivity. To be vulnerable, personal, emotional, even tender became not only acceptable but desirable in the new masculine mystique. Women found this softer image attractive and sexy. He-man ballplayers, long-distance runners, and tennis stars reflected the changing social trends as they honed their sales skills in commercial endorsements. It was the age of unisex and "doing your own thing." Under contract to beauty firms and appliance makers, mustached jocks grew their hair long and blew it dry in the locker room and on television screens across the country. A big breakthrough occurred when three famous New York Yankee tough guys—Joe Pepitone, Yogi Berra, and Hank Bauer—held up a can of hair spray and said, "I'm no sissy and I use my wife's hair spray." Earl "The Pearl" Monroe, of the New York Knicks, took the lead in the fashion parade with his eye for good tailoring. And men all over were opting for denim suits and gold chains, and taking off those extra pounds.

In the past ten years, stars of the sports world have pushed everything from hair products to colognes to underwear; even Joe Namath sold pantyhose on TV, and who would dare call Joe Namath unmanly? Much to the credit of these athletes, men who took care of their appearance no longer bore the stigma of narcissism and effeminacy. Unisex, divorcing fathers obtaining custody of their children, and a new awareness of man's potential for a fuller range of emotions have become acceptable. At last a man has permission to indulge himself in what was once only a woman's privilege: a sensible preoccupation with good grooming.

It was only a matter of time until men would begin to pay attention not only to their physiques and their clothes, but to their complexions. The Egyptian king Tutankhamen was buried with cosmetic jars, and in Beowulf's time men dyed their mustaches green and blue. Today, moisturizers and other skin-care products, as well as salon facials—once strictly the province of women—are being bought by more and more men. It's now okay for a man to say, "My skin also gets dry and sometimes there are breakouts and a tendency to acne." Where once he may have borrowed his wife's or girlfriend's eye cream and hand lotion, today a man is no longer reticent about buying skin-care products made expressly to enhance his appearance.

It's a dynamic new decade. Everywhere you turn today, diet and exercise programs are being offered to keep our bodies young and supple. The means to expand our youthfulness have never been more varied. With this new awareness, cosmetic surgery for men has come of age.

As we enter the eighties, there is an increased acceptance of plastic surgery for purely cosmetic reasons. And the plastic surgeon treats not only the physical but also the psychological needs of his male patients. The role that the plastic surgeon plays is being recognized as a positive one in the medical world and in society.

This book has been written for those of you men who yearn for more, who want to live your life to its ultimate potential, who may have the need for new opportunities. If you are entering a new relationship, contemplating a career change or a move up the corporate ladder, and notice changes in your face that might be affecting the way you as well as others view you, then now is the time to reappraise your situation, concern yourself with your goals for the future, and perhaps consider any improvements you can make through plastic surgery. Of course, age is no barrier. Cosmetic changes are possible at forty and still acceptable at seventy. It is never too late. When is the best time? When it's the right time for you.

Cosmetic surgery is no longer the exclusive property of the rich and those in the public eye. It is not only our best tool for correcting nature's more visible mistakes—such as a cleft palate or a disfiguring nose—but it can also be an attractive solution for wrinkles, drooping eyelids, undereye pouches, sagging chins, crepey necks, and the ravages of advancing years. Until recently, women have had an edge on men in their relation to cosmetic surgery. It was always more socially acceptable for them to have plastic surgery. No more. The times are changing. Now, men, too, are visiting plastic surgeons' offices, determined to reduce the effects of premature aging and, in some cases, deciding to correct those imperfections that they had reluctantly accepted all of their lives.

We live in a new era where chronological age is not a true barometer of how we feel or look. Most individuals who lead active, healthy lives just don't seem to age as quickly. Better nutritional habits, advanced medical techniques, diet, exercise, and the invaluable psychological need to think, to look, to feel younger—all work together for our collective and individual benefit.

But then, suddenly, seemingly overnight, the mirror reflects a new visage, one that has definitely aged. Nothing we can do can permanently hold back the years. When that happens, why shouldn't a man consider keeping his face and body in tune with how he feels? Why not cosmetic surgery? After all, if a man in his fifties feels and participates like a thirty-year-old, isn't he somewhat at a disadvantage if he doesn't look the part?

Looking good used to be almost the monopoly of the "beautiful people," those who had the money and the time to fly off to the latest spa to lose a few pounds and to try the newest exotica in a series of rejuvenation shots. These youth worshippers went south for hush-hush eye-lifts and a tuck here or there. And of course Hollywood's heroes have a vital economic reason to take care of those signs of aging. Their careers depend on looking young for as long as possible.

But what happens when an average middle-aged man looks into the mirror and is suddenly dismayed to discover that, after lessening the bulge around his middle, the bags under his eyes are even more conspicuous than before? His face just doesn't match his body—or his self-image—any more. Perhaps more calamitous is the aging executive, still full of drive and ambition, who fears being passed over for an important promotion in favor of some younger, less experienced man. His sixty-year-old face masks his thirty-year-old attitude, and can unfairly affect his future.

It happens far too often. A man may have attained great prominence, achievement, and financial success, yet he will still feel insecure if he glances in the mirror and sees the wrinkles, pouches, and lines that emphasize the many years that have passed. It is the same for a recently divorced man who has to reestablish himself. He must keep his spirits up, reorient his goals, and learn how to make it on his own. He may want to have another go at romance, but his face threatens to undo his high hopes. It's a downer.

But today there is hope for such men, who now account for as much as 20 to 30 percent of the cosmetic surgery performed in this country. And that figure is rapidly increasing. Face-lifts, eye-lifts, and hair transplants are being done, and some men are choosing to have nose corrections, ear reductions, and reconstructions of the body as well.

Men have finally discovered that there is no reason to live with the mistakes of nature, or to sit by and permit the aging process to detract from a still-vigorous body. It is no longer unmanly to be "vain"; in fact, a certain amount of vanity is considered a healthy step in raising one's self-esteem. With today's new, improved techniques of plastic surgery, and the new climate conducive to change and self-improvement, men have their first real opportunity to look their best and to look younger longer.

Quick and inconspicuous operations, performed in doctor's-office complexes, have made it easier for more men to turn to cosmetic surgery as a solution to premature signs of aging. Not as much time is expended nor as much money spent as, say, ten years ago. There is also less need to go public about one's decision—a man doesn't have to be out of his office long enough to elicit unusual questions, or to make up excuses. For those individuals who prefer to keep any cosmetic work confidential, a vacation or business trip can conveniently cover the time period necessary for any visible bruising to diminish, although there should be no reason to be ashamed of having had surgery or to conceal its aftereffects.

The greatest change in plastic surgery today is the type of candidates themselves. Until fairly recently, plastic surgery attracted a select group of men—those in the theater, TV, or Hollywood; male models, and other public figures. Many of the men opting for surgery now come from the mainstream of society: teachers, lawyers, blue-collar workers, stockbrokers, even priests and rabbis. Men who seek cosmetic changes today cover the entire spectrum of our society. As each procedure has gained wider acceptance, we find that there are fewer emotionally insecure, unstable personalities who must be eliminated as potential candidates. Unfortunately, there are some men whose expectations are so unrealistic that no amount or type of plastic surgery changes can satisfy them; the psychological and emotional trauma that can result in these situations prevents physicians from accepting them as patients.

Some experts have expressed doubts that cosmetic surgery can really make any major difference in one's life. I feel, for instance, that the benefit of a face-lift is a psychological as well as a physical one. When a man's emotional state is elevated, when he's feeling more positive about his appearance, he usually takes better advantage of whatever opportunities he meets. As a matter of fact, I have been told so often by so many of the men I have operated upon that their lives did change significantly, that it seems obvious to me that the psychological effects of cosmetic surgery are more far reaching than the physical result. Perhaps it won't win you the job you want or save a broken marriage, but its emotional benefits are more often than not real and positive.

For example, one forty-six-year-old patient of mine, Robert J., confided to me that he was insecure about his status in his corporation. After being with the firm for more than twenty years, Bob had decided to have a face- and eye-lift. Later, he told me that it was worth far more to him than he had initially realized. A few weeks after the surgery, Robert was contacted by an executive-search firm on the West Coast. Feeling confident and relaxed about himself, he accepted a new and higher paying position with a rival company within six months of the initial contact.

The psychological benefits of cosmetic surgery are varied. For some men, it permits them to be more aggressive; for others, to exhibit more confidence; and for most, a feeling of being "refreshed," "better," "neater," "more youthful." These are just some of the comments I hear over and over again from men describing their emotional moods during their postoperative visits.

Is it vanity that compels men to seek cosmetic changes? Most men today seem unconcerned with the question. The macho-for-macho's-sake image has subtly but constructively evolved into a more wholesome one; if you look strong and radiate health and youth, then that is what is considered manly today. Many men used to enter my office under assumed names, acting furtively, as if they felt ashamed to be there. Today, they phone for appointments with no embarrassment or need to resort to subterfuge.

Men are feeling better about themselves, collectively and as individuals. Men ask more technical and in-depth questions regarding the surgery. Being specifically concerned with the placement of incisions and the resulting scars, they're in general more self-conscious about having the surgery done than women. Motivated by the same needs and desires as women, to look better and feel more confident, their expectations are generally realistic; they don't expect to turn the clock back thirty years. The very fact that men are coming into the office in increasing numbers and actually undergoing the procedures indicates the change in attitudes of men in relation to themselves and plastic surgery in the 1980s.

With surgery costs no longer prohibitive, as well as being legitimate tax deductions, more men can afford the procedures. Improved techniques, equipment, outpatient facilities, and available surgeons have all been factors that have helped to lower prices and bring cosmetic surgery within the financial reach of the average man. And the average man is taking advantage of it.

I sometimes find myself referring to plastic surgery as "psychosurgery" because of its deep involvement in the psychodynamics of image alteration. To be effective as a plastic surgeon, I must work very closely with my patients, both before and after surgery, not only on the physical aspects of the procedures, but also on their emotional consequences.

First, I discuss with each prospective candidate the procedure's possible complications and its effects and alterations, on both the physical and psychological level. I always examine and evaluate the patient's motives for, and expectations from, surgery. If his expectations are unrealistic, and I feel that the surgery will not solve his more deeply rooted problem, then I advise against it. I base my decision on an evaluation of the total picture—the man and his motives—and then use my judgment as to whether or not I can achieve what he hopes for. For example, a forty-eight-year-old man who decides that his overly large ears cause women to reject him may be overreacting to one small defect and not facing other possible causes. If the focus seems narrow or misdirected, the individual may be unconsciously choosing an insignificant problem and using it as a rationalization for a more serious disturbance in his emotional makeup. Repeated failed love affairs, a deep conviction that he is not attractive to the opposite sex, combined with approaching fifty, might have contributed to a continued depressed psychological state that has very little to do with the size of his ears. His problems may best be evaluated by a therapist and not a plastic surgeon.

What makes a man decide to have cosmetic surgery in the first place? We really can't generalize that easily about motivations—they differ from case to case: a man who has recently been divorced and is now actively dating; a man who feels that a more youthful look may be beneficial to his business; a man who may simply be unhappy with the way he looks and has finally decided to do something about it. There are many reasons why men come to my office to seek cosmetic surgery. But what we can agree on is that cosmetic surgery is that specialized area of medicine that one elects to have; and it almost always comes from the desire to make a positive change. Even in the case of a car accident, where the victim's scars might be unsightly, only when the individual wants to have the scarred site treated is a plastic surgeon sought.

Most often, a candidate for cosmetic surgery has a healthy premise for having a procedure done. When the need for correction is sensible and real, and within the realm of what I, as a surgeon, can do, I take the candidate on as a patient.

Cosmetic surgery is an elective procedure. It should be chosen by basically healthy patients who can safely tolerate anesthesia, be it local or general, and whatever surgery is to be performed. If there is pain or discomfort, it is only temporary. The plastic surgery patient is usually more relaxed, knowing that he has chosen to be uncomfortable for a short time for the sake of being better off in the long run. It's a tradeoff, and most of my patients know and accept it. The word "suffering" is not a valid description of the experience. Remarkably, even the more anxious patient feels relaxed during the post-surgery period, often saying something like, "It was as easy as having my hair cut."

"External" and "Internal" Motives

Whether the particular problem is obvious or imperceptible to others may not matter to the man who is considering surgical correction. What is important is the way he views himself. In our society, attractiveness is prized. A high premium is placed on physical attributes. Because of this, whether or not we agree with the value system, individuals are often judged by their appearance. Often they are their own severest judges. Interestingly enough, in a recent study conducted of three-year-olds in Canada, psychologist Karen Dion found out that this young group had already formed firm opinions about their attractive and unattractive peers. The better looking you are, the better off you may be. Not only are attractive people presumed to be more successful in business, they are also presumed to be kinder, warmer, more sincere, and more sociable than more homely people. While this is a broad generalization, as my own practice indicates, more and more men are agreeing with this.

Although I do not conduct a formal psychological test on the men who come to my office for a consultation, I do form an opinion of both the man's demeanor and his requests. If his appearance seems normal, his behavior not extreme, and, if during our discussion his reasons for wanting surgery seem within normal range, as do his expectations, then I would consider him an appropriate candidate. Of course, many questions are asked, on both sides of my desk, that help me make a sound judgment. You'll find some of those questions and answers in chapters 3 and 4.

The male menopause may also affect a man's motivations. Although men obviously do not go through the same physiological stages that women undergo during this time of life, many profound psychological changes do occur. Headaches, erratic changes in behavior, quickly shifting moods, and decreasing libidinous drives are some of the symptoms that may occur during the male menopausal state. There can also be stress, sleep disturbances, and depression—anywhere from mild to severe—in the older male. If I feel that a man who consults with me about changing his appearance is mildly depressed, I will discuss alternative therapies with him; for example, psychological counseling. I will advise him that although I can reduce the flab under his chin and remove his eye pouches, I can't cure his depression through surgery. However, very often the results of a face- or eye-lift may make a positive difference in the emotional state of a man experiencing an identity or age crisis.

Accidents can severely maim or scar, leaving a damaged personality. For a burn victim, there is a great adjustment to be made. Studies have been done on how and why physically disabled or sick people behave as they do. The results indicate that all patients do not adjust on an equal basis. Some are overly compliant while others are uncooperative. All of this research, appearing in medical journals, is helpful to me as a surgeon. I must keep abreast of the latest findings so that I can be well informed on how to assess and treat each individual who comes to me for consultation. I also must often stimulate motivation for recovery—an interest in getting well—for those individuals, such as burn and cancer patients, who need special restorative plastic surgery work. Scars, disease, severe burns, and mutilations can adversely affect the personality so that such a severely disfigured person loses the will to fight—and often the will to live.

Some patients come to see me with what turn out to be very minor problems: barely noticeable scars or minuscule wrinkles. I am usually leery of such people. They won't be happy, no matter what I do for them. Not every scar needs to be erased, nor every line or wrinkle removed: they give character, distinction, and often sophistication to one's appearance.

I recently saw a man in his early twenties who requested that the very fine lines about his eyes be taken away. I found it peculiar for such a young man to be so concerned with an extremely minor problem. What will happen to him when he develops additional signs of aging? It will cause a crisis. He may be the type of individual who rushes in almost yearly for whatever minor corrections he thinks need to be made. I refuse such cases, as most surgeons do. His motivation isn't healthy enough, and his expectations are unrealistic. This is exactly the type of patient who would be unhappy about the work if a doctor did accept the case, no matter how excellent the result.

Most of the patients I see are reasonable, mature, and sensible. It is, in fact, rare for me to come across anyone who is obviously psychologically disturbed. An individual must have a fairly healthy ego to want to improve himself in the first place. The truly emotionally disordered person doesn't have the ability to see what improvements he might want to make. But when I do encounter a prospective patient who seems severely neurotic or even psychotic, poorly motivated, and dishonest with me and himself about what he really feels or expects, then I flatly refuse to operate.

Of course, I want to do good work, to help those in need, and achieve a pleasing result. But even the most successful face-lift sometimes falls far short of the expectations of the man who secretly wants to resemble Paul Newman. I cannot change the basic structure, the expression, the personality behind the face, and I tell every candidate I see that it is important for him to recognize right at the outset that we are skilled doctors who want the best for our patients but are not gods who perform miracles. For after all is said and done, plastic surgeons are people, too.

TWO

Plastic Surgery: Then and Now

PLASTIC SURGERY is by no means a modern phenomenon. There are references to its techniques both in the Bible and in other ancient sources, such as Egyptian papyrus fragments that date back to about 3000 B.C.

In those ancient times, long before the invention of the printing press and today's even more sophisticated means of communication, surgical techniques were often confined to one geographical area, and, within that region, to only one or two family members. There certainly was no community of surgeons. Today, of course, if there is an advance in, say, microsurgical techniques in a Danish medical center, the procedure is observed and written up in professional journals that are disseminated throughout the world. And when they choose to, surgeons from almost anywhere on the globe may fly to a particular medical center to see for themselves the new procedures being performed. Because of this revolution in communications, medical technology spreads quickly throughout the world. Knowledge becomes cumulative, with one surgeon making improvements on the techniques of another. Nonetheless, the surgeons of ancient times, working in isolation, and without knowledge of anyone else's activities, often did remarkably sophisticated work. Ancient man practiced trephination (boring holes in the skull) as a crude form of medical treatment for certain illnesses, hoping it would release evil spirits. The Babylonians, during the time of Hammurabi, 1950 B.C., performed an operation for removal of cataracts of the eyes. In fact, when the records of such procedures have been discovered, modern-age surgeons have realized that there was much to be learned from them.

• • •

ANCIENT SURGERY

The first plastic surgery we know of involved reconstruction of the nose. In ancient times the nose was more than just the organ of smell; it also had symbolic value that related to manhood and virility. (As a matter of fact, in some cultures, we still talk about a "manly" nose.) When a warrior wanted to show off the prizes of his victory, he didn't flaunt only gold from looted villages; often he exhibited sliced-off noses that once belonged to the captured enemy. While this practice sounds, and indeed is, barbaric, it nonetheless has continued through contemporary times in some civilizations. And so it is easy to see how a physician with the skill to reconstruct a nose could be a very valuable asset to a community.

Reconstructive surgery—especially nose reconstruction—had its beginnings in India. The cosmetic art has actually been practiced on that subcontinent since at least the seventh century B.C. At that time the earliest descriptions of surgical techniques in India were written by a surgeon named Sushruta. Sushruta can, with justification, be called the father of modern plastic surgery, because he is the first known physician to describe the transplantation of skin—the key element of plastic surgery as we know it.

The writings of Sushruta describe many operations, including reconstruction of amputated noses and the removal of cataracts. They also tell in detail of such procedures as removing gallstones, performing Caesarian sections, and more. Even the surgical instruments are described.

Both commerce and conquest transmitted Sushruta's methods to the ancient Greek culture. Hippocrates, the father of Greek medicine, more than likely was aware of Indian surgical techniques. Sushruta's works were translated into Arabic in the eighth century and into Latin in 1844.

However, it has been puzzling to many scholars why knowledge of the Indians' medical achievements should have been unknown to Europe for so long, particularly considering England's close involvement with India since the early seventeenth century. It wasn't until 1794 that a letter to the editor of a general-circulation English periodical called *Gentleman's Magazine* made Europeans aware of what had been happening in India since Sushruta's time. The letter

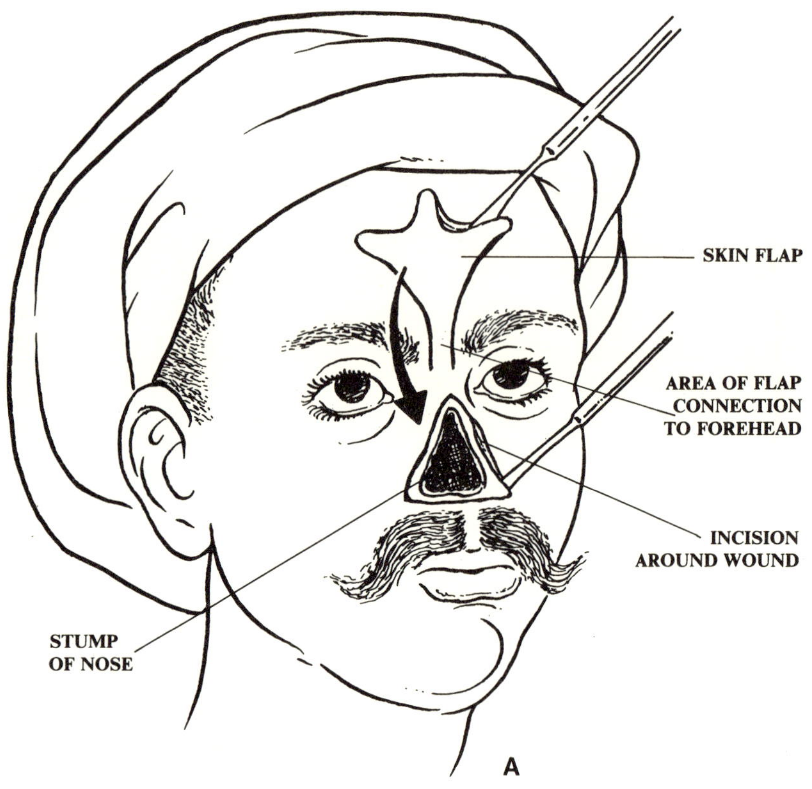

Indian Nose Flap

described how a reconstructed nose was affixed to a man's face by a member of the brickmaker caste near the city of Poona.

The method of restoring the nose, now known as the "Indian" method, used skin from the patient's forehead. First, a plate of wax was formed into the shape of a nose. It was then flattened and placed on the forehead. A line was drawn around the wax and the surgeon dissected as much of the forehead skin as was covered, leaving uncut a small slit between the eyes. This slit allowed the blood to circulate until the skin was sutured into its new position. If no blood were to circulate, the skin would die. When the skin was

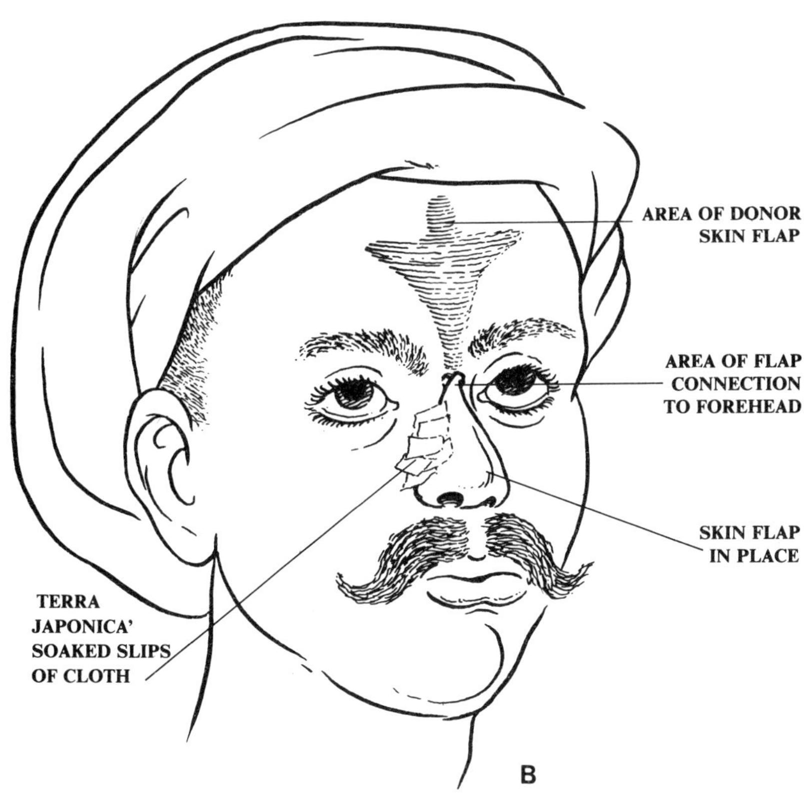

brought down from the forehead, it was turned in such a way as to create a new nose.

This type of operation was successfully performed in 1814 and 1815 by the English surgeon Joseph Corpue. He copied the Indian technique for two nasal reconstructions—one operation made necessary by the patient's misuse of mercury that was prescribed to treat a jaundice condition; the other by a battle wound. Reconstructive nose surgery was afterward performed by other surgeons of the time. And so, ironically, it was not for many centuries that Europe finally caught up with the scientific skills of one of its colonies.

EARLY SURGERY IN EUROPE

During the early 1400s, a Sicilian surgeon named Branca successfully performed nasal reconstructive surgery. Historical records indicate that his skills were passed on to disciples, including his own son, who apparently used skin from the patient's arm rather than from his forehead. This technique became known as the Italian method, to differentiate it from the Indian method.

Throughout the 1500s, similar surgery was performed by members of the Vaineo family in a small town near Calabria, Italy. Chances are that the Vaineos were unaware of the work performed by the Brancas. It is important to note that, at this time, the actual number of surgeons who practiced plastic surgery was never great and generally was concentrated in one area.

In the late 1500s Gaspare Tagliacozzi contributed much to the popularization of plastic surgery. A professor of anatomy and medicine in Bologna, he left for posterity descriptions of all the surgical techniques then known in Italy that involved reconstruction of mutilated parts of the body. Ironically, after Tagliacozzi's death, there was very little plastic surgery performed in Europe for a period of about 200 years. The surgical art fell into disrepute, and was not taken seriously by the medical profession.

There were some surgeons who did consent to help patients who needed reconstructive surgery during the years when plastic surgery was in decline. But most of them remain unknown today. In the early nineteenth century Carl Ferdinand Von Graefe was a renowned teacher in Berlin when he was not traveling with the army as director of medical operations. One of his outstanding surgical achievements was a successful operation that closed a cleft palate. He also made contributions to nose surgery, performed cataract operations, and partially resected a lower jaw.

In the 1820s the German surgeon Johann Diefenbach developed techniques to repair clefts of the hard palate. He also did reconstructive work on the nose, ears, lips, and eyelids, as well as pioneering restorative work on many parts of the body, from clubfeet to elbow joints. Diefenbach was also the first in Germany to introduce ether as an anesthetic agent.

MODERN SURGERY

In 1898 Dr. Jacques Joseph, an orthopedic surgeon in Berlin, reported his first rhinoplasty operation. This operation is important in the development of plastic surgery because it was the forerunner of what we know as cosmetic surgery. It did not involve the reconstruction of a nose disfigured by disease or accident, but rather a nose that was esthetically too large. The patient simply wanted its size reduced.

Dr. Joseph was able to transform the nose without leaving any scars. He did this by getting at the bone from within the nostrils. In his published papers Joseph described such procedures as the removal of nasal bumps and the shortening of a nose.

The procedure was revolutionary, and so was the concept of "cosmetic" surgery rather than surgery for life-saving purposes. As a result, Joseph had to try hard to convince his colleagues that the type of surgery he performed was medically ethical. To some degree he succeeded. In retrospect it is easier to see Joseph's ultimate success because his work has been developed and refined through the years. His name is in the forefront of pioneers in plastic surgery.

Pioneering work in jaw surgery was performed by American surgeon Vilray Blair early in this century. His photographs, probably more convincingly than his words, showed the medical community the amazing work he had accomplished in, for instance, correcting the abnormal positions of the chin.

The work of men like Dr. Blair, particularly those surgeons who performed so heroically and expertly during World War I, did much to bring plastic surgery into good repute among doctors and the public. Blair himself was chief of plastic surgery for the American forces in Europe in 1917 and 1918.

When Blair returned to the United States after the war, he established the first plastic surgery unit at Barnes Hospital and Washington University in St. Louis. In 1921 he helped found the American Association of Oral and Plastic Surgeons. The surgery performed on facial injuries and burns, for example, was far too important to ignore or consider superficial. And what was learned during the war had its applications even during peacetime.

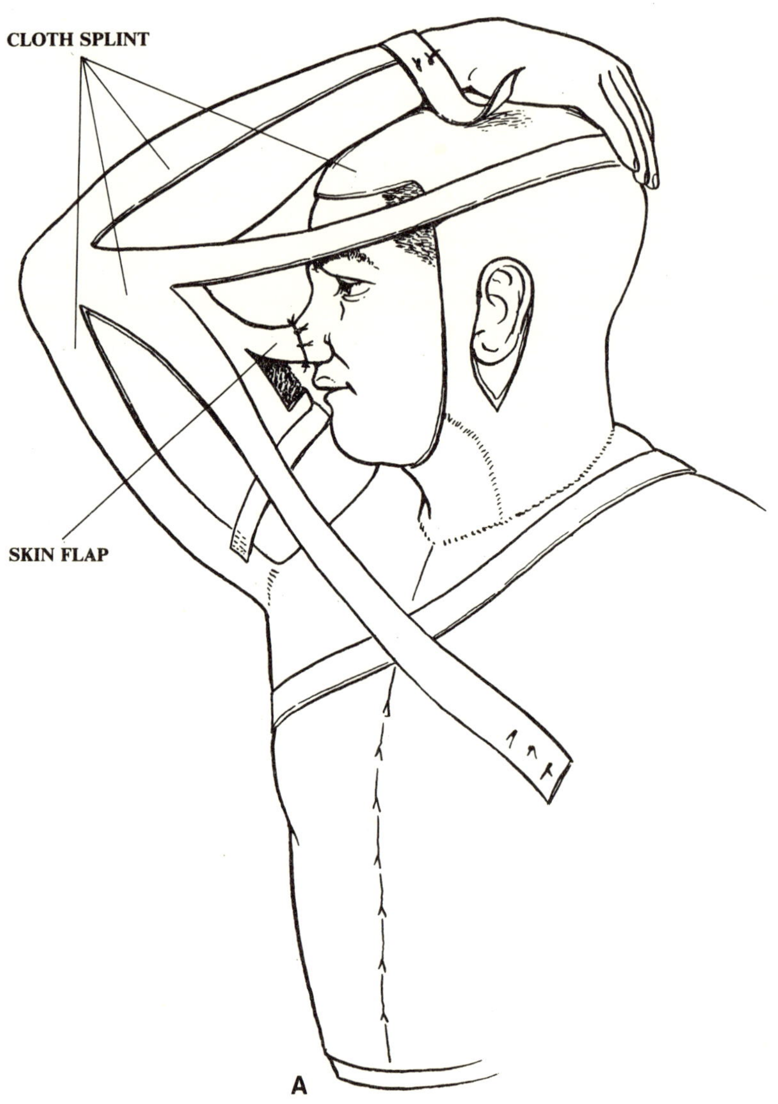

Tagliacozzi Arm Flap

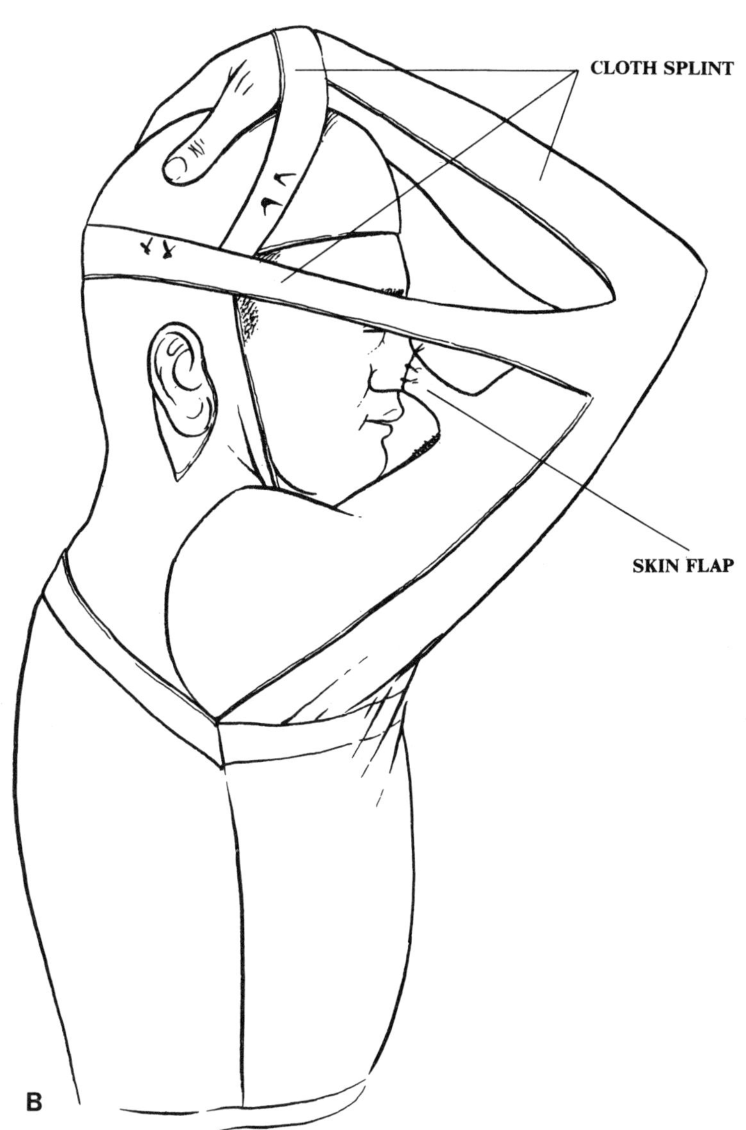
CLOTH SPLINT
SKIN FLAP
B

There are many other people who have contributed to the art of plastic surgery as we know it today—too many to name. Men and women working at this very moment will be cited in the textbooks of tomorrow. Many more surgeons will be known for their skills with the scalpel, and medical engineers will become famous for the new tools and machinery they will develop for these surgeons. From microsurgery to new procedures and tools, progress continues in plastic surgery. There are many more exciting chapters to be written.

SURGERY TODAY AND TOMORROW

By observing current trends in plastic surgery, it is possible to look with some degree of accuracy into the future. For example, as we already know, the number of people electing to have cosmetic surgery is increasing rapidly, almost to the point where it is as common as having one's teeth capped. This means that in ten years there will probably be many more than the 2,100 board-certified plastic surgeons who are practicing today.

Similarly, there will be even more outpatient facilities in the future, and therefore less need to go to a hospital for most procedures. Since most people would rather avoid hospitalization, more men and women who were once hesitant will be willing to undergo cosmetic surgery. These outpatient facilities will also be located throughout the country, making it less necessary for someone to go to a metropolitan area for surgery.

It is difficult to say where the medical breakthroughs will be, but there are certain promising areas that are receiving a great deal of attention. Microvascular surgery is one of them. Microvascular surgery is the technique for repairing small structures that have not been adequately seen before. The lighting and high magnification of modern microscopes, together with fine micro-instrumentation and microsutures, have enabled us to repair small structures with a precision heretofore not possible. Medical wonders are being performed right now, as amputated parts of the body, such as cleanly severed hands, arms, or fingers, are reimplanted through microvascular surgery. An increasing number of surgeons is being trained in this field, and there are more and more medical centers where such operations can be performed. Unfortunately, not in every instance will implantation be attempted. The amputation must be clean-cut; there can be no crushing of a serious nature; and the amputated member must be placed in an ice solution and rapidly transported to the medical center that happens to perform this type of operation.

There was publicity for the microsurgical work performed at Bellevue Hospital in New York after a young music student had her right hand amputated as a result of being pushed in front of a subway train. Here, there was a relatively clean cut, the dismembered hand was placed in an ice solution, and there was an experienced staff at Bellevue to undertake the long and intricate operation, which successfully reimplanted the hand.

This operation consists of anastomosing blood vessels that are only two millimeters in diameter. This means resuturing the severed ends of the arteries and veins involved. The painstaking procedure takes a long time—as long as twelve hours. So delicate an operation is possible only because of microscopes that can magnify nerves and blood vessels up to forty times their size. The microscopes are connected to a television screen, enabling the rest of the medical team to see what the chief surgeon is doing. The tools that are needed in the operation—the tiny scissors and forceps, and the extra-thin surgical thread—are important elements in the operation, along with the skill of the surgeons. Follow-up is important in this type of surgery because some of the reconnected blood vessels can close down and require reoperation. All in all, it is a time-consuming, delicate procedure requiring great skill on the part of the surgeons and support personnel.

Within this field of microsurgery, a great deal of experimentation is also being done with free tissue transplantation. This involves the process where we take a section of skin, frequently with underlying muscle and even bone, and place it somewhere else on the body. The key here is to remove, along with the skin, the vessels that carry the blood supply. A skin flap the size of a pancake four to six inches in diameter can therefore be taken from the groin area and sutured, along with its blood supply, to vessels in the facial area where reconstruction is necessary because cancerous tissues were excised.

This procedure, which is being performed in more hospital centers, usually requires only one surgical step. Without it, it would take multiple surgical procedures for the reconstruction to be completed.

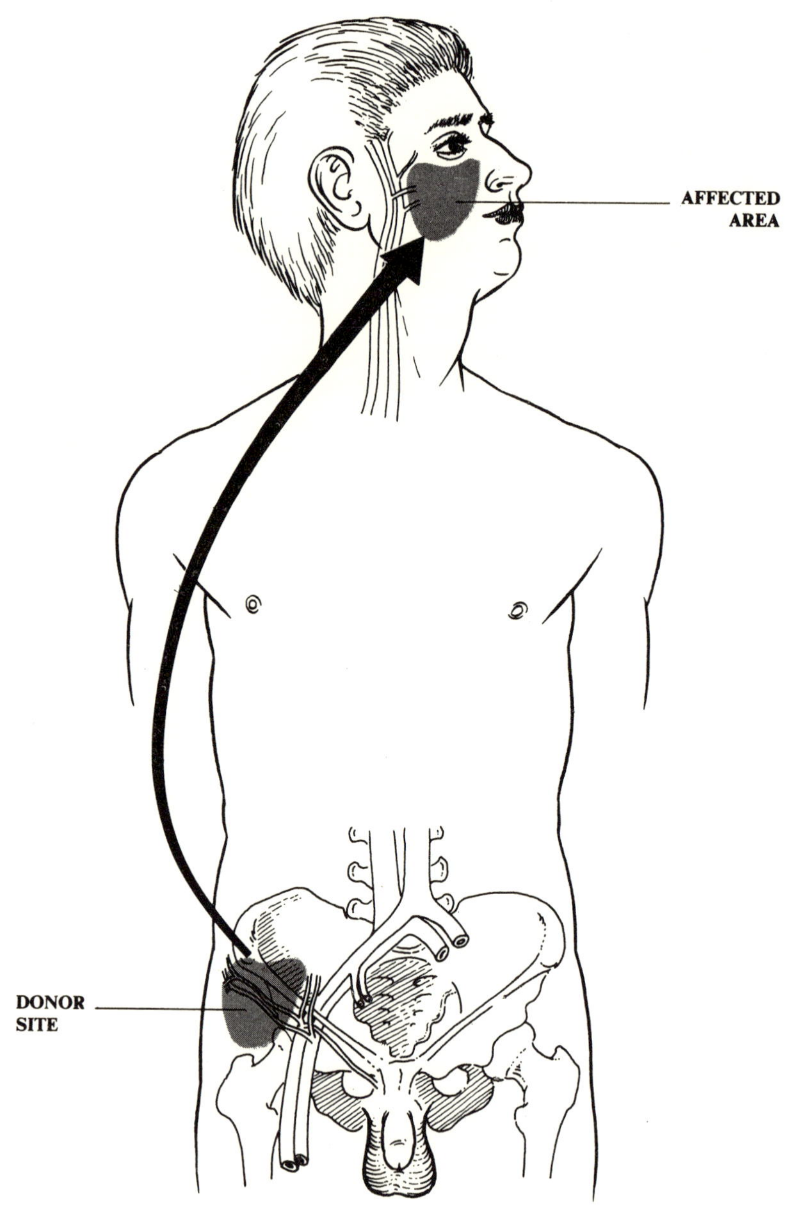

Groin Donor

Right now the work is being done mostly in university hospitals and training centers for residents in plastic surgery.

Microsurgery has had other applications, not as widely publicized. For example, an esophagus removed because of cancer can be replaced with a part of the patient's own intestine. Partially paralyzed faces have gained mobility because of microsurgically transferred nerves. In the event of an aneurism within the brain (an aneurism is a weak spot in an artery, which may rupture, leading to a stroke, or even death), the aneurism can be removed and the tiny blood vessels resutured through microvascular techniques.

In many quarters there are excellent expectations for surgical breakthroughs with laser-beam technology. While the laser, as yet, has not been the miracle surgical tool that some of its adherents claim, there is still a great deal of experimentation to be done, and in another ten or twenty years there may be many more successful laser applications. For instance, the laser beam has been used in removing skin discolorations such as port wine stains, and has had limited application in the removal of tattoos. It is currently a surgical tool in eye surgery to seal detached retinas and to use in treating certain tumors of the larynx or voice box. Future uses may include wider applications and further advances in surgery in all these aforementioned fields.

Increased attention is being given to the treatment of the 300,000 serious-burn victims who are hospitalized each year. More facilities and more surgeons are specializing in burn treatment. In addition to using the patient's own skin for grafting purposes, experimentation is being conducted with pigskin, amniotic or fetal membranes, and a variety of other biological dressings which are being studied for the possible use in treating burn patients.

In the medical journals and through other professional channels, there is a steady stream of reports on advances in surgical procedures. Not all of them, of course, have application for plastic surgery. Yet we read and we learn—and in some instances we can adapt one of these new techniques. Cardiovascular radiologists at Johns Hopkins University Hospital, for example, have created a balloon made of silicone that is allowed to travel with the blood in the vessel. When the balloon is in place it is inflated so that it fits in the vessel snugly. The balloon thus acts like a tourniquet. The developers of this technique see it as an easy way of preventing excessive bleeding during surgery, particularly after accidents.

Plastic surgery is involved to a large degree with altering the inevitable change of the aging process. But why we age and how we can live longer will continue to be matters of conjecture and research within many disciplines. Not only will we continue to research and work in such specifics as preventing hair loss, but there will be studies and applications done on how, in general and specifically, we may retard the aging process through better diet and overall healthful lifestyles.

The breakthroughs that we will see within the next decade or two will not necessarily come from the United States. Or, for that matter, from Western Europe. For example, while many people think a great deal of plastic surgery is performed in the Scandinavian countries, perhaps because of the notoriety caused by the Christine Jorgensen sex-change operation, actually very little cosmetic surgery is done there. In Russia, however, where one wouldn't expect much cosmetic surgery to be performed, there are long lists of patients awaiting doctor's appointments. Plastic surgery research is also being done in China, Japan, and the East European countries.

Besides being transmitted in professional journals, ideas are also exchanged at meetings and seminars. I have often traveled to foreign countries to observe new techniques and procedures being performed. It is a part of a plastic surgeon's work and when I can make time I find such meetings, dialogues, and exchanges educational and valuable as a means of improving my skills as a surgeon. In the future there will be more use of videotapings so that surgeons will be able to observe the various new procedures without traveling.

There is no doubt that there will be many advances in the field of plastic surgery. We live in a marvelous age where satellite television, closed-circuit monitoring of operations, and lightning-quick communication help us all to become aware and stay aware of developments in the field. It's an exciting, ongoing, and dynamic branch of medicine.

THREE

How to Select a Plastic Surgeon

When you have your car repaired, you want an expert mechanic. When you get your hair cut, you seek the most skilled barber. It stands to reason then that when you are considering something as important to your well-being as plastic surgery, you want not just a good plastic surgeon; you want the best one around.

There are millions of Americans who undergo some kind of plastic surgery each year. How do they find their surgeons? They select them in many ways, and not necessarily scientifically. If you are contemplating plastic surgery, you shouldn't rely on random luck in choosing a qualified doctor. Here are some suggestions on how to go about selecting the right surgeon for the job.

Ask for qualifications. No surgeon should be upset when you ask about his qualifications. Today's doctor doesn't expect to be treated like a god; he will be more than happy to give his *curriculum vitae,* which lists his training, his education, his special honors, and his hospital affiliations. He may tell you his qualifications, hand out a sheet that reports them, or even give you a personal guided tour of his office, where you will notice at least one wall that contains his diplomas and other certificates and honors.

Look for board certification. When a plastic surgeon is "board certified," it means he is a member of the American Society of Plastic and Reconstructive Surgeons. Before he becomes a member he goes to college, spends four years in medical school, a year of internship, and at least three years of general surgical training, after which he does specialized work in the plastic surgery field for two years. The specialized plastic surgery training is accomplished within one of the approximately 100 programs approved by the American Board of Plastic and Reconstructive Surgeons.

At the end of the two-year specialty period, the surgeon is "board eligible." This means he is qualified to take his examinations. First there are several hours of written exams. Approximately a year after these exams the surgeon presents before a board of plastic surgeons cases that he has worked on independently during his time in private practice. He must also take an oral examination given by the examiners of the board.

So when you go to a plastic surgeon who has "board certification," you can be assured that he has spent a certain number of years training in his specialty and has passed examinations given by his peers. Not all plastic surgeons who are certified are equally skilled, of course. But they all have fulfilled at least certain requirements and must have evidenced a degree of competence to be judged members of the board.

There are approximately 2,100 board-certified plastic surgeons in the United States; the numbers are increasing at the rate of about 150 to 200 a year. A book that may be in your local library lists all board-certified specialists in the country. Called the *Directory of Medical Specialists,* it is published by Who's Who, Inc., 200 East Ohio Street, Chicago, Ill. 60611. All board-certified surgeons are listed by their specialty, their state, education, training, and membership in professional organizations. If your surgeon is certified he will be listed in the directory.

Get recommendations. It helps to know of someone who is familiar with the quality of work performed by the surgeon whose services you are considering. A friend who has had plastic surgery may recommend a surgeon to you, or your physician may be able to give you the name or names of qualified surgeons.

Check accreditation. The surgeon you choose should be on the staff of an accredited hospital. That's because such a doctor is constantly being judged by his surgical peers. If the doctor were to have problems in a hospital, he could be called before the hospital's medical board. There are cases where doctors have been removed from hospital staffs because their work did not meet standards.

Hospitals also check on their staff doctors to make sure that they are taking all necessary courses and are keeping up with the latest technology, as, for example, the requirement to attend a course in cardiopulmonary resuscitation. The American Board of Plastic and Reconstructive Surgery and other specialty boards see to it that members are kept up to date on all developments in the field through dissemination of professional publications. Recertification is being required in many specialties.

To find out if your surgeon is with an accredited hospital, consult the book *Joint Commission on Accreditation for Hospitals.* If you have any questions about your surgeon's competency, you can contact the American Board of Plastic and Reconstructive Surgeons, Inc. 29 East Madison Street, Chicago, Ill. 60602.

HOW TO MAKE THE MOST OF YOUR CONSULTATION

The consultation is very important to you and your surgeon. It's the time when you get to know the surgeon and he gets to know you. You will want to use this time wisely and not walk away saying, "I wish I'd asked him a few more things." You're a step ahead if you've read up on the procedure beforehand. The fact that you are reading this book shows that you rightly want to know as much about the procedures available from as many sources as possible.

Before you visit the doctor's office, prepare a list of questions you would like answered. What do you have doubts about? What aren't you sure of? If you don't have everything on paper, you're likely to forget something because of anxiety or nervousness.

A question you may want to ask is: "Is plastic surgery for me?" Many patients come into the office, but they aren't sure whether they need surgery. The surgeon will honestly tell you whether, and to what extent, you will benefit from surgery. At the first sign of a wrinkle, for example, you may run to a surgeon for a face-lift, only to be told that you should wait a few more years. Or you may want a hair transplant when there is not enough hair to fill in the bald spots effectively. (See chapter 4 for the twenty-six most common questions patients ask their surgeons.)

COST AND THE RECOVERY TIME

The cost and the recovery period are two matters that concern every man who contemplates plastic surgery. Unfortunately, medical insurance rarely picks up the costs, so what you invest will probably come out of your pocket. Any extended recovery period where you have to miss work can also cost you money, so determine the total costs and be sure you are willing and able to spend the money before you make a commitment.

The exact costs cannot be estimated to the penny, for fees vary from surgeon to surgeon and even to some extent from state to state, city to city, and neighborhood to neighborhood. The recovery time also varies, from patient to patient—some men are just faster healers than others. With that warning, here is a range of figures for various procedures, along with recovery time.

Hair transplant. If the procedure uses plugs (a cylindrical section of hair-bearing scalp) the fee would depend on the number of plugs that are transplanted. Fees range around $10 to $15 a plug, and as many as 500 plugs may ultimately be needed.

Eyelids. The fee for eyelid surgery runs from $1,200 to $2,000. Recovery generally takes from a week to ten days. After two weeks the patient can return to work even though there may be some slight swelling and possibly minimal discoloration.

Face-lift. When the operation includes the neck as well as the face, the fee could run from $2,000 to $4,000. If the face is done in conjunction with eyelid surgery, the range is from $3,000 to $6,000. Recovery period is about two weeks.

Nose. Fees are from $1,500 to $2,500. The cast doesn't come off for about a week. It usually takes another week before you are comfortable enough to return to a full schedule.

Body contouring. Breast reduction to correct male gynecomastia (enlargement of breast tissue) costs between $1,000 and $2,000. A two- to three-day hospital stay is usually required as well as a seven- to ten-day recovery period.

The fee for abdominal lipectomy (removal of redundant fat and skin from the abdominal wall) ranges from $2,000 to over $3,000. There's approximately a two-week recovery period, and four to five days in the hospital.

Chin and jaw. This would depend upon whether a simple implant was used or more complicated work on the mandible was involved. A simple implant costs from $500 to $800, while for more involved procedures the range is $1,200 to $4,000. Recovery time is a week for implants and much longer for complex surgery.

Dermabrasion (a mechanical method frequently used to correct post-acne scarring). Fees run from $800 to $1,500. Recovery time is approximately two weeks.

A SURGEON'S SPECIALTIES

Plastic surgery is a specialized practice of medicine. But there are even specialties within this specialty. There are plastic surgeons who are known for doing hand surgery exclusively. Others will do only reconstructive surgery, and still others practice only cosmetic surgery.

The work of most plastic surgeons, however, is more varied. If the surgeon has been in practice for a while, chances are he may gravitate toward the cosmetic-surgery field. He may no longer want to run from hospital to hospital handling emergencies, as he did when he started out. At that point he may get a junior associate. There are many, both newcomers and veterans, however, who do cosmetic surgery as well as the equally challenging reconstructive surgery.

OUTPATIENT FACILITIES

Advanced techniques, rising hospital costs, a decrease in the availability of hospital beds, and an increased demand for more plastic surgeons have all contributed to today's increasing trend toward cosmetic surgery on an outpatient basis. Many cosmetic-surgery procedures are not covered by insurance policies and so, in order to care for patients at a reasonable fee, many plastic surgeons have opened up their own private outpatient facilities.

What surgery may be safely performed on an outpatient basis? Procedures such as face-lifts, eye-lifts, nasal surgery, and minor cases of male gynecomastia can all be approached in this manner; while such cases as abdominal lipectomy or the reduction of a large breast are probably best handled in the hospital.

Not all people are good candidates for outpatient surgery. For instance, if a patient comes to me with a cardiac history, or a medical history of unusual bleeding, or if an elderly man has medical problems, I might recommend operation in a hospital setting. Generally, though, this is not the case. I often see individuals in their sixties, who are in good health and have no serious cardiac or pulmonary problems, and can therefore have cosmetic surgery on an outpatient basis. Most of these procedures are done using only local anesthesia.

Selecting candidates for outpatient surgery can be determined during the initial consultation. It's important to note that the patient experiences no more pain or discomfort if he is operated on in an outpatient facility than he would in a hospital. An outpatient setup is equipped for administering medication to diminish any operative discomfort (although obviously not as strong as that given in-hospital). Patients walk out of outpatient facilities under their own power. The minimal amount of discomfort encountered during surgery is adequately covered by medication administered during the surgery. After a period of rest, the patient can return to the comfort of his own home.

The prospective patient should ask questions about the facility and may also want to see the actual operating room. Any accredited surgeon will have the proper facilities and backup; still, one should remember to be diligent about checking the surgeon's credentials, his affiliations, and the facilities in which he operates. Surgeons with their own outpatient facilities will be happy to show these to you.

In the usual outpatient procedure the patient is kept on a stretcher in a waiting area, where the premedication is administered prior to surgery. From this stretcher, the patient is taken for the surgery to the operating room. After the operation he is placed back on the stretcher and taken to a bed in the recovery room.

This procedure is exactly the same as that of a hospital, but my own opinion is that the patient receives more attention on an outpatient basis. First of all, the staff is specifically trained to handle cosmetic-surgery patients on an everyday basis. They are, therefore, more apt to spot any potential problems, should they arise. As for me, I feel more comfortable in my own facility because I have a staff I work with every day, and I am familiar with all the equipment and instruments. Greater efficiency results from such a situation.

The outpatient facility will also have an adequate dressing room for the patients, a waiting or pre-operative area for holding before surgery, and, as already mentioned, a recovery room. The operating room does not have to be particularly large but it should be well organized and of course clean, with walls and floors that can be

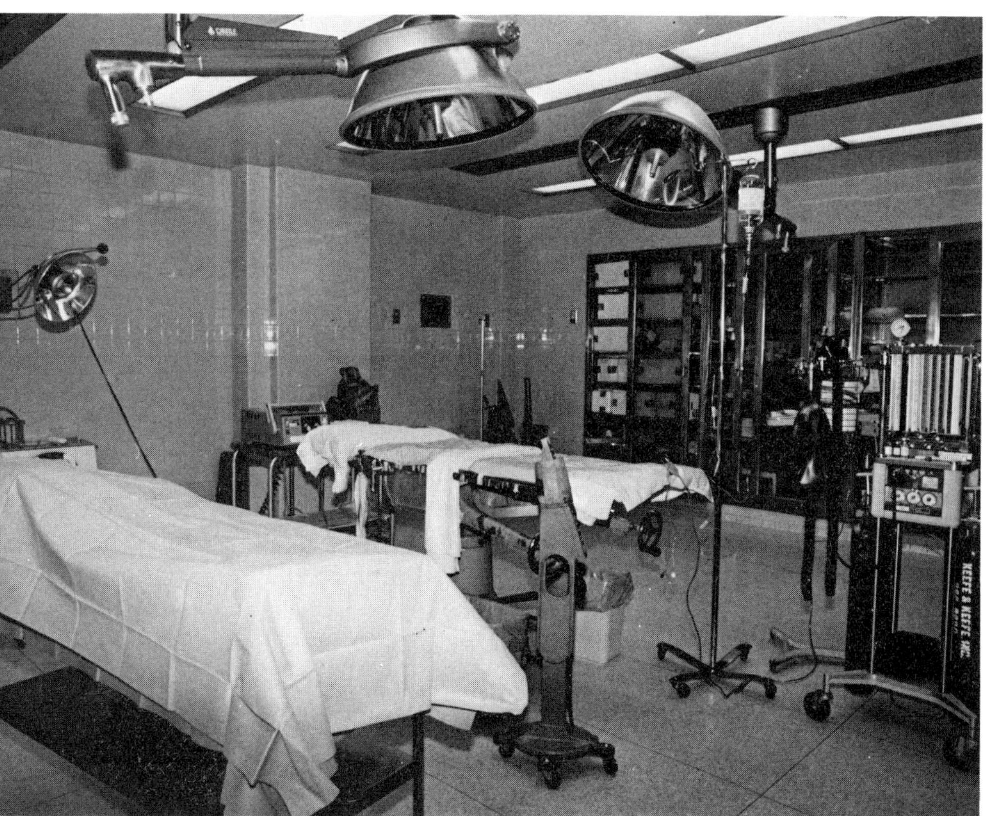

The operating room

washed easily between each surgical case. There should be a wash-up area where the surgeon can scrub up before surgery.

Soon after the patient is brought into the operating room, an intravenous is started; this establishes and maintains a method of administering any medications to be given during the surgery. In those rare instances of minor reactions to medications, the effects can be readily reversed through the intravenous route. All the equipment and medications necessary are at hand. Attending at the operation is usually one assistant to the surgeon, as well as a scrub nurse who can not only hand the instruments to the surgeon but assist in holding and retracting them during the procedure. There is also another nurse or medical assistant circulating in the operating room, in case additional instruments or supplies are needed. This last person allows for more efficient operating-room functioning. Usually, only one surgeon works on a patient at one time. Frankly, when one is working on the eyes, the nose, or any feature of the face, two doctors would get in each other's way. We use the same masks, caps, sterile gloves, and gowns—all the equipment that is used in a hospital. Instruments are sterilized in an autoclave before each case. Those of us who have our own operating rooms must meet or exceed the standards required by a hospital. And we do.

If you investigate the surgeon and you feel he is qualified, then more than likely his personnel are also qualified. A doctor is out for the best possible results for the patient; he is not going to jeopardize his reputation or the outcome of the case by working with inferior help, or in substandard operating-room conditions.

Some surgery is performed under general anesthesia, but for most male cosmetic surgery local anesthesia is used. Surgery is usually carried out in the morning and early afternoon, when everyone feels the freshest. In the later afternoon, I see postoperative patients and have new consultations. Most of the patients operated on in early morning are ready to go home by early afternoon.

A patient usually waits about an hour before the actual surgery, which takes from one to three hours, depending on the specific procedure. Postoperatively, there is usually a two- to three-hour recovery period. Since most outpatient surgery is done under local anesthesia, and the patient is not heavily sedated, we advise prospective candidates who will not tolerate the slight discomfort attendant in and after the surgery to select an in-hospital setting. Some people cringe even at the thought of a needle.

What happens if an emergency arises? I insist on and conduct routine staff drills every few weeks, during which time potential problems are simulated and dealt with. At present time there are no jurisdictional agencies controlling private doctors' operating rooms, but as more and more OR's spring up, various regulatory organizations will get more involved in the establishment and regulation of standards. More local and federal regulations are in the offing.

• • •

IN-HOSPITAL SURGICAL CLINICS

Many major hospitals and teaching institutions maintain clinics for patients who cannot afford the standard plastic surgical fees. Such prospective candidates are seen and evaluated by a senior member of the staff. The surgery is usually performed by one of the plastic surgeons who is in training. What this means is that the doctor has completed medical school, has at least three years of surgical training, and is either in his first or second year of a training program in plastic surgery. It's helpful to realize that clinic patients are not operated on by just anybody and that all procedures are supervised by a board-certified plastic surgeon.

It is explained to the patient that he will be operated on by the resident physician under strict supervision. For this reason, fees for clinic services are usually less than those charged by private physicians. There are clinics that are maintained by some of the major teaching hospitals in the country. Depending upon your financial position, you might want to investigate one of them. Remember that the advantages of having a private physician are that you get ongoing care and see the same doctor all the time. The responsibility for your surgery rests with your operating surgeon.

The major plastic-surgery procedures performed at clinics are hair transplantations, face-lifts, eye-lifts, and nasal surgery. These are routinely performed under local anesthesia; however, patients are frequently admitted for one- to two-day stays. The cost of this stay will frequently be subsidized by the hospital as part of its resident training program. Such hospital clinics serve as a good source of patient material for the resident.

POSTOPERATIVE CARE

Once the operation is over, a patient will frequently have specific questions about the surgery he has just undergone. Most often, he will ask advice on how to minimize the postoperative side effects he will experience.

In the first place, one of the things I always tell the patient is that most people won't even realize that plastic surgery has been performed. Patients occasionally have guilt feelings about having had surgery performed, and some become almost paranoid; they think that everyone is looking at them now that they've had the surgery, and they become quite self-conscious. In point of fact, most of your co-workers will not notice that anything at all was done to your face when you return to work. You may hear comments like "Gee, you look refreshed"; "You look better"; "It looks like you've had a good vacation." But that's about all.

You may be concerned about some slight discoloration around the eyes if you've had eyelid or nasal surgery, or some discoloration in the facial area after facial surgery. However, by the use of some very simple tricks, many of these temporary telltale signs can be covered up. Here are some helpful cosmetic hints for various surgical procedures.

Hair Transplant

The patient who has just had a hair transplant, and has had hair plugs taken from the back of the scalp and placed in the front, will find that the scalp requires some cleaning up for two to three weeks, as a result of old crusted blood. Within two to three days after the transplant, the dressing is removed. At that time, I usually suggest that the patient take a shower and use a very mild shampoo on his scalp. Vigorous scalp massage is not recommended for at least two weeks, because it can loosen the plugs. Some patients may be a little disturbed the first few days after surgery because the hair will be matted down with old blood and tissue fluid; however, with careful shampooing twice a day, the hair will soon be cleaned out. It can then be carefully blown dry, using the cooler temperature of the dryer, and patients can then restyle their hair in such a way as to cover up the healing areas. Most patients who have had hair transplants are particularly knowledgeable about styling their hair before the transplant surgery, and they certainly know the best way to cover up the operative sites.

Face-Lift

For the patient who has a face-lift, I usually recommend, in the pre-op consultation, that he plan to let his hair grow a little bit longer than before. I don't expect a man in his fifties to make a sudden, radical change in his hair style, but I do advise skipping the barber for a two- to three-week period before the surgery, allowing the hair to become a bit longer. In the postoperative period it can then be combed to camouflage the incision sites.

Another question most frequently asked is "When can I wash my face?" Thorough cleansing of the face and scalp can be beneficial in removing the dried blood that may remain in the hair, and helps keep the operative site clean. The dressings and the drains come off after approximately twenty-four to forty-eight hours, at which time—as mentioned above—I tell the patients to shampoo their hair at least once a day, and, if they wish, lightly blow-dry it on the dryer's cool setting. Naturally the patient should avoid vigorous use of the comb and brush, to avoid entangling them in a suture. If this should occur, the suture should not be pulled but gently dislodged from the comb and/or brush.

After the operation I suggest that the patient sleep with an extra pillow under his head. It is difficult of course to control the positions that people sleep in, but I find that patients are acutely aware of the surgery, and usually lie flat on their backs for the first few postoperative days. Incidentally, turning in various positions will not appreciably alter the effects of the surgery (assuming that the patient has an extra pillow under his head). The elevation of the head has a tendency to reduce the edema, or swelling. For the first few mornings after surgery the patient may notice a fair amount of swelling, but as the day goes on and he stands erect, this decreases significantly. For those men who dye their hair, I recommend that they do not use the dye for at least two to three weeks after the surgery, or until the incision sites are healed.

Eyelid Surgery

Using ice compresses for the first forty-eight hours is beneficial in the immediate postoperative period. Although continuous application of ice is difficult, even intermittent applications of cold compresses can not only be soothing to the eyes but can substantially reduce the swelling. In the postoperative period some patients occasionally develop an irritation of the eyes; this is explained by the fact that because the redundant skin of the upper lids and/or lower lids has been removed, the corneas are going to be slightly more exposed. In certain industrial areas or big cities, where the air contains a fair amount of particles, the patient may notice irritation or redness of the eyes; for this condition, I usually order any of the over-the-counter eye drop preparations. Rarely does the condition become more involved; when it does, I prescribe medicated eye drops.

The simplest way to cover up any postoperative eye discoloration is to use dark sunglasses, either mirrored or the regular type. You may want to have one or two pairs of glasses when you go back to work. You may choose a slightly tinted pair if you want to return to work only a few days after surgery. Such lightly tinted glasses won't draw as much attention to you as a very dark pair. I tell each of my patients that whether he is one of the fastest healers or one of those who may develop considerable discoloration, everyone tends to look good within ten days to two weeks.

Nasal Surgery

Many of the patients who have had nasal surgery wonder how soon they may take a shower because of the cast that is applied. I have no objection to their taking a shower within a day or so following surgery, as long as they don't get the cast wet. The cast is there to protect the nose, help reduce the swelling, and hold the repositioned bones in place: if it comes off prematurely it may affect the result—and wet casts can come loose. If a patient wants to wash his hair, it would be best done in a bathtub, leaning the head back rather than having the water in the shower run down the face and onto the cast.

Eyes become swollen after nasal surgery, and the routine use of ice packs, for twenty-four to forty-eight hours, helps to reduce swelling. After forty-eight hours I see no reason to continue using the cold compresses, either for facial, eyelid, or nasal surgery, because the swelling reaches its maximum at forty-eight hours and then recedes by itself. Ice is probably not beneficial after two days. As the swelling of the postnasal surgery resolves itself, the cast may become loose, at which point I tell the patient to just retape the area with adhesive tape. The patient may feel uncomfortable with the cast while walking on the street, but it is usually off in five to seven days after surgery, at which point the patient will feel less self-conscious. If there is some discoloration around the eyes, sunglasses can be used. They should not rest on the nasal area but should be taped up to the forehead. I do not suggest the wearing of heavy glasses, but when glasses are necessary, they should be worn so they don't rest directly on the bridge of the nose.

Ear Surgery

The dressing is left on for five to seven days after surgery. Frequently patients are advised to let their hair grow long before the surgery. Most people who have ear surgery have usually worn their hair long anyway because of self-consciousness about their ears. I advise that they shouldn't switch suddenly from a long hair style to a short hair style. I suggest a slow hair style elevation, revealing the ears by degrees. The long hair style will camouflage the new ear shape or position, and changing the hair style slowly will not draw attention to the surgery. I also suggest wearing a ski band around the head and ears at bedtime for the first few months. It avoids the problem of lying directly on the ear and gives confidence, protection, and security in the postoperative period—the patient doesn't have to worry about his ear being bent accidentally while sleeping. If the band falls off in the night, it probably result in any damage to the operative area.

Abdominal and Breast Surgery

Camouflaging is not really so necessary after these procedures. The dressings and drains are usually off within a few days and, because of the area of surgery, clothing will cover everything. After two to three weeks, most of the discoloration and swelling in the chest area are gone. The sutures are all removed and the small incision in the infra-areolar area is almost invisible. I would suggest that these patients protect themselves at the beach and avoid direct sunlight and sunburn for the first three weeks following surgery. Approximately three to four weeks after the surgery, they can start to increase their exercise and work on a suntan. Surgery done in the breast area around the pectoral muscle can cause some tenderness, so avoid vigorous exercise for the first few weeks.

In doing an abdominal lipectomy, we frequently firm up the muscles at the time we remove the extra skin and fat, so there can be some slight discomfort in the abdominal area. I do not recommend that patients do extensive sit-ups or calisthenics for at least six weeks after the surgery, particularly if there has been extensive muscle suturing in the firming up of the tissues. This does not preclude patients starting to jog two weeks after surgery and slowly building up their tolerance for exercise.

FOUR

The Questions I Am Most Frequently Asked

NO ONE goes into surgery blithely and totally assured that everything will turn out well. There is bound to be some apprehension. But there is one type of anxiety that is unnecessary—anxiety caused by ignorance. Man fears what he doesn't know. That is why I encourage my patients to read about plastic surgery and then to ask me any questions that are on their minds. Although what I am asked varies from individual to individual, there is nonetheless a common thread. Many of the same questions are in the minds of nearly all my patients. Here are the most commonly asked, along with the answers I generally give:

General Questions

I feel terribly awkward and out of place here. Aren't most of your patients women? And actresses and society women at that?

There are an increasing number of men who are realistically seeking plastic surgery. They're not oddballs, either. They're normal businessmen, white- and blue-collar workers, men from all walks of life. In the last five years of private practice I have helped a great number of men who have become aware of what plastic surgery can do for them.

Is it going to be painful?

No. Cosmetic surgery is not painful because the area worked on can be numbed with novocaine—what the dentist uses; we couldn't operate if you felt pain. And on the day of the operation you won't be apprehensive—that's because you'll be given sedation before surgery.

Is it dangerous?

As in every surgical procedure there are problems and unforeseen side effects that can occur. But serious and truly dangerous effects are extremely rare.

If the operation doesn't turn out well, will I look worse than before?

No, but the end result you had hoped for may not be fully achieved. Each operation has a limited purpose; it is designed to do only one thing. Let's say after surgery on your nose there is still a small residual bump. It can be removed in a second minor procedure. Let's also consider the situation of eyelid surgery—after it's over, all the bags under your eyes might not be completely removed. Here, too, a second procedure can usually solve the problem. Incidentally, there's usually no charge for such revisions—that's because your surgeon wants the best result possible both for you and for his own sense of pride and professionalism.

Hair Transplantation

Should I get a hair transplant or settle for a toupee?

If there is only a small amount of hair on your head, you may not be a candidate for surgery. There's not enough hair to shift around. If you were just beginning to recede in the forehead area or had only a balding pattern at the top of the head, and yet had a fair amount of hair on the back of your head, you would be a candidate for a transplant. In most cases, the patient with limited, sparse hair would be best advised to consider the alternative of a toupee, or just to accept the baldness.

When will I be able to get back to work after a hair transplant? And how long do the dressings have to stay on?

You should be out of work for only a few days. A rearrangement of existing hairs should cover some of the operative scar sites, particularly at the back of the head. There will be some scabs for about ten days, however, so you may want to wear a light gauze pad with a hair piece over it, or, merely adjust the existing hairs over the healing plugs.

Will the newly transplanted hair fall out?

Yes, the hairs fall out in two to three weeks and then slowly regrow. These usually last the lifetime of the patient. (This will be described in chapter 5.)

Eyelid Surgery

Is eyelid surgery dangerous?

No. The incidence of complications is very small. Discoloration is to be expected and resolves itself quite rapidly. Vision is not impaired though some blurriness may occur as a result of the eye solution placed in the eyes at surgery—this subsides in a few hours.

Will I have a "starey" look?

There's no reason why you should. If a conservative amount of skin is removed from the upper lids and smaller amounts of skin and fat from the lower lids, you should have a normal appearance about the eyes. Any wide-eyed look will resolve itself when the swelling goes down. Obviously there is some "open eyedness." The purpose of the operation is to remove skin—reduce hooding and remove excess skin of the upper lids and puffiness of the lower lids. You will have a look that is refreshed, less tired, and very natural.

Will my eyes be more sensitive after surgery?

Yes, because they will be slightly more open than before. Pollution or high atmospheric-particle density may also cause a temporary chemical conjunctivitis or irritation of the cornea. A mild eye ointment or solution recommended by your surgeon should take care of the problem.

What about my contact lenses?

After surgery to correct excess skin of the upper lids and/or puffiness of the lower lids, contact lenses shouldn't be used for about ten days, but can be readily worn thereafter.

Nose Surgery

How will I breathe if there is packing in my nose?

Packing does not have to be placed in the nostrils after surgery. Whether or not your nose is packed, there probably will be a fair amount of swelling and crusting of old blood on the inside of the nose for at least a week, and this will inhibit breathing to some degree. At the end of the week, breathing freely through the nostrils should be easier. Breathing through the mouth is not difficult—you've done it many times without effort when your nose has been stuffed from a head cold.

Will I be black and blue?

Yes. There will be a fair amount of discoloration and swelling around the eyes because the surgery involves working around the loose tissues around the eyes and nose. A small amount of blood will be discharged through loose tissues of the eyelid area, causing the discoloration. The swelling is the reaction of the tissue to the surgery.

How long will the cast be on?

For about one week. You will be advised to apply cold compresses to your eyes for the first few days, to help bring down the swelling.

What will I look like when the cast is off?

There will still be considerable swelling. But with the cast off you'll be able to see improvement, since any undesirable feature or bump will be gone. The final result won't be observed, however, for several months. But you can return to work within two weeks—a good deal of the swelling will then be down.

What about bleeding?

There will be some oozing from the nostrils after surgery, but it usually stops within a day or two. Heavy postoperative bleeding is unusual, but if it does occur it can be arrested with packing and cold compresses applied to the nasal area.

My breathing is impaired because of a deviated septum. Can the blockage be cleared up and my appearance improved at the same time?

The procedures are frequently combined in a one-stage operation, so the obstruction from your septum can be taken care of while cosmetic improvements are made to the visible portion of the nose.

Face-Lifts

How long will I be away from work?

You should be back in the office within ten days to two weeks after a face-lift. You'll feel relatively comfortable and look much improved. A change of hair style, a new growth of beard, or a mustache may be used, if you like, to throw colleagues off guard. Ideally, being away for ten days to two weeks will give you enough rest, combined with the surgery, to give you a refreshed look on your return to work.

When can I start shaving?

Since the facial sensitivity will be somewhat increased, use an electric razor for the first seven to ten days after surgery. You may, however, want to grow a beard for a few weeks after surgery. A beard is a good way to divert attention from the fact that there has been surgery.

Is it true that you use drains in the face-lift operation?

A drain is used to collect any blood that might accumulate under the skin as a result of the surgery. This minimizes swelling and helps prevent postoperative complications, such as blood accumulated beneath the skin. A dressing is also used, and it remains for about two days. It keeps the swelling down.

Is there a way to hide the black-and-blue marks?

Within a week or ten days the swelling and a good deal of the discoloration will be gone. If any black and blue remains, there are special powders and lotions that I will recommend to cover up and soften any bruised look.

How can I cover up the scars?

The face-lift involves incisions, and therefore scars, in the hairline above the ear and behind the ear. It's a good idea to let your hair grow longer before the surgery so that you can easily cover up the scars. When they are fully healed they should be relatively inconspicuous, although you should recognize that no surgery is performed without scars. A slight alteration of your present hair style will allow you to be comfortable while the incisions are healing.

Do I have to change my diet after the operation?

Only for the first couple of days, during which time you should be on a soft diet. This is the period when your face will feel a little tight; but within forty-eight to seventy-two hours you should be able to resume your normal eating habits.

When can I resume jogging and swimming?

After about ten days to two weeks a good deal of the healing will have taken place, and you can start jogging and doing other exercises. But start out slowly because your face has been operated on and part of the healing process involves an increase of blood flow into the area. Strenuous exercises will further increase the flow of blood into the area and might cause some discomfort. After three or four weeks you should be able to resume most of your normal activities, including sports.

When the stitches are removed—a week or ten days after surgery—swimming can usually be resumed. If any areas of the wound are superficially open, however, they may be irritated by salt or chlorine in the water. And if your eyes have been operated on in conjunction with the facelift, swimming should be avoided until several weeks after surgery.

Breast Reduction

How long will it be before I can exercise and participate in sports?
The stitches around the nipple are usually removed within ten days after the operation. In the first few days there can be some postoperative discomfort because of the proximity of the underlying pectoral muscle—as well as the relatively wide area of skin undermined. After about a month you should be able to resume most of your normal activities. The operation takes place at a level above the muscle so that the ability of the muscle to function is not affected.

Dermabrasion

Will dermabrasion remove the crow's feet by my eyes?
Not every line can be removed by eyelid surgery (blepharoplasty). Crow's feet cannot be removed, but the horizontal lines around the eyes may be softened somewhat by an abrasion.

THE TEN MOST UNREALISTIC REQUESTS

Most men who come to my office are fairly sophisticated about what the field of cosmetic surgery can and cannot accomplish. The press and other media have devoted much space to the subject, and so most people today are already aware of the procedures and have seen some rather famous faces displaying the results. Nonetheless, there are still some who do seek the impossible—what, for lack of a better term, we might call a miracle. Often, a life crisis may have recently occurred—the death of a loved one, the loss of long-standing employment, or a divorce, which may deeply affect the individual so that he wants to make radical changes in his life and in his appearance, expecting those changes to fill up the lack, the empty areas that may now exist. In these cases, supportive therapy may be the answer, while cosmetic surgery should be put off until the person is sure of what he really expects any procedure can do for his life.

When a prospective patient wishes for an unrealistic result and his consultation with me leads to other problem areas, I explain the limitations of any surgical art, for no surgeon is a magician. I want to make sure that the man is going to accept these limitations before we proceed with any surgery. Otherwise, he might very well grow more disturbed after the operation than he was before.

By presenting the following typical questions about plastic surgery that I consider to be unrealistic, I don't mean to imply that you shouldn't ask about anything that is on your mind, even if you fear sounding foolish or naive. It's imperative that you find out what the operation involves, how much it will cost, how you will look and feel afterward, and what the results are apt to be, along with any possible complications. And you can only find out whether your expectations are realistic by sitting down, talking openly with a doctor, and asking him whatever you feel you want to know.

I'm seventy-five years old. I would like to think that I could pass for much younger, like forty-five. Is this possible?

In a total face-lift procedure, which would involve eye-lift and neck as well as face, there will be considerable improvement. The skin is elevated, drawn back, and the excess excised. You will look better and no doubt younger. But you are unrealistic if you expect that you can take off as much as twenty or thirty years. Even if the procedures were to remove almost all of your wrinkles—and this is by no means assured—there would be other indications to your age. Your expression and your posture, for example, are subtle signs of age that are natural. What you should strive for is to look refreshed—less tired and aged—to be content with looking better and not looking thirty years younger.

My face is unlined, except for the lines that are prominent from my nose to the corners of my mouth. Can they be removed?

The nasolabial—or smile—lines, cannot be obliterated totally, nor should you want them to be. You should realize that this is a normal facet of the human appearance, and that expressive lines are natural. In some cases, an inherited characteristic for deeper, more pronounced nasolabial lines exists. Silicone injections can soften them somewhat, but it is not a procedure that I usually recommend. The face-lift procedure will soften the lines but cannot totally eradicate them.

It's very difficult for me to stay on a diet. Would a face-lift give my face a slimmer appearance?

A good result can be achieved only if you lose any excessive weight before the surgery and get to your ideal weight. It's impossible to remove fatty deposits from a face that is really fat because of an overweight condition; it is the excess skin and excess fat in specific areas, such as under the chin, that can be taken away, but the entire face cannot be thinned out. And after all, what about the rest of the body?

Since my wife passed away I've taken more care of myself and paid more attention to my appearance. I have excess facial skin; it sags, and that bothers me. Can an operation tighten it up?

Yes. However, one operation will improve the condition, but more than likely you'll need a secondary one because of your great amount of excess skin and its laxity. Since you are in your sixties and you haven't had surgery before, the first procedure can tighten the skin, but there will be some postoperative stretching. A secondary operation, about a year or sooner after your first face-lift, should maximize the result. Certain men need the benefit of a second lift; this doesn't mean that the first isn't successful, but merely that some individuals get a maximum benefit from two lifts.

I hear that you can cut away fat from my abdomen to give me a slim profile.

You hear wrong. Fat cannot be cut off. You first have to lose the weight. If, after this, the remaining excess skin sags, then this flab can be surgically removed.

I'm sure I'm one of your best patients. And a satisfied one. You've improved my eyes, face, and neck, and I'm delighted with the results. But now, what about my hands—the loose skin and discolorations on top—can you help me here?

Here's where I can't help you. The results are unpredictable. While plastic surgeons repair congenital abnormalities as well as acquired injuries, removing discoloration or tightening up loose skin on the hands would leave scarring, which would be worse than the initial problem, and it is not routinely done by most plastic surgeons. You have to draw a line as to what you can expect from plastic surgery. Now's the time to start drawing it.

Doctor, I'm thinking of having my stomach done. I also noticed a new wrinkle this morning on my face and it made me sick—it has to be taken care of.

You've had everything possible done and apparently you're still unhappy with yourself. I'm sorry, but further surgery—another face-lift or other procedures—will not make you content. You look fine. Perhaps you should seek the causes of your discontent within yourself. Surgery isn't the answer to everything. Therapy might be a help to you now, to look a bit closer at where you feel you are in your life, how you relate to others, and how you feel about yourself.

I know I could have landed a particular television part if I had a dimple. I understand plastic surgery can create one. Can you do it?

In my experience, attempts to place dimples in the chin have generally been disastrous. It's impossible to get a natural look. Most results look more like an excavation of the face. You are good looking; why take a chance of ruining those looks? Besides, do you really think the absence of the dimple was the cause of your losing a part?

I have a tattoo on my arm. Once it had a reason for being. Now, it's a source of embarrassment. Can you remove it?

So far there is no completely satisfactory procedure for removing tattoos. There has been some talk about laser techniques but as yet the results are not predictable and they are still not widely used. The appearance of the tattoo may be softened, but the outline will remain. The area can be cut out and a skin graft can be placed there, but the area will be depressed and a scar will replace the tattoo. Also, skin corresponding to the area of the tattoo will be a different color after skin grafting, so that the results will still be far from ideal.

I would like a natural hairline. I understand that hair plugs and other techniques can accomplish it, but I have only a thin rim of hair. Can this still be done for me?

Surgical techniques can transplant hair from one area of the scalp to another. But in your case it can't be done, simply because you don't have enough hair to begin with. You need more than a thin rim of hair to achieve any degree of success in hair transplantation.

PART TWO

The Procedures

FIVE

Hair Transplantation

As many as 80 percent of all men can expect to experience some hair loss during their lifetimes. In fact, as they age, women as well as men will lose some of their hair, for hair loss is a normal physiological process. It is only when the loss is irreversible, when hair doesn't grow back and the scalp becomes visible, that the situation can be traumatic or disturbing. The technical name for baldness, whether in a male or female, is alopecia. When it occurs in a relatively young man, hair loss leading to baldness can be a blow to the ego. There is a certain mystique of virility about a man's head of hair, and how much or little he has may influence how he views himself.

The truth is that no matter how common hair loss may be, few men adapt to it, all sense some sort of deficiency, and many mistake it for a lessening of sexual power. Hair is a sensuous part of the anatomy; it is tended to daily and it changes with the dictates of fashion and time. But rarely does the shiny pate of a Yul Brynner or Telly Savalas inspire imitation.

One of the theories about hair loss is that it is caused by genetic predisposition, which may come either from one's paternal or maternal side. Nevertheless there are many cases where the individual may be the first one of his family to experience male-pattern baldness.

The onset of baldness is usually a gradual process; the hair-producing follicles begin to function less and less. Biopsies have been taken from various parts of the scalp to determine whether there is any difference between the hair-bearing and non-hair-bearing areas; aside from a thinning of the epidermal layer of the skin in the balding areas, there is no histological pattern or difference that can be discerned under the microscope between the two areas. The hormonal pattern in baldness is also still undetermined. Some researchers have suggested the use of androgens—male hormones—to reverse the process. Dihydrotestosterone (DHT) is a potent androgen at the cellular level, and it is thought that it might be helpful in the prevention of balding. Nevertheless, studies and application have so far proved inadequate and DHT's role in preventing baldness is yet to be resolved. Even though there have been recent news reports that a Chinese doctor, using a combination of herbs, has effected new hair growth, such tests and studies are still in the preliminary stages. For now, it remains a case of genetic predisposition. There is also no proof that the male-pattern baldness is related to either too-tight scalp muscles, mental stress, too much or too little shampooing, or local skin conditions. Although there are many theories on the subject, the cause of baldness is still unknown.

From my standpoint as a physician, the psychological loss that often accompanies hair thinning, and which can parallel aging, may create emotional problems, and in some cases damage otherwise self-assured images, in the patients I see. Men have been known to use everything—from false hair to makeup, to penciling and stenciling on the semblance of hair shadows, to mask a balding head. The results have never proved satisfactory. Hair transplantation, a relatively new medical procedure, can often help and may provide a more natural and lasting solution.

Not only skin, but also more complex structural components can be transplanted from one part of the body to another, with a reasonable assurance that the transplant will survive in its new location, provided certain medical and basic surgical techniques are practiced. We all are familiar with the remarkable work done in skin grafting: a severely burned patient's skin can be taken from one part of the body and transplanted to the burned area. If this area is properly prepared, the newly transplanted skin can be expected to grow. It is this innate ability of the human being to accept certain tissue from one part of the body to another without rejecting it that is the basis for hair transplantation.

Opposite page: Typical progressive balding pattern with advancing age. Male pattern baldness can begin either in the front or on the top of the scalp. More commonly it is a combination of both, eventually resulting in the typical "horseshoe" fringe of hair.

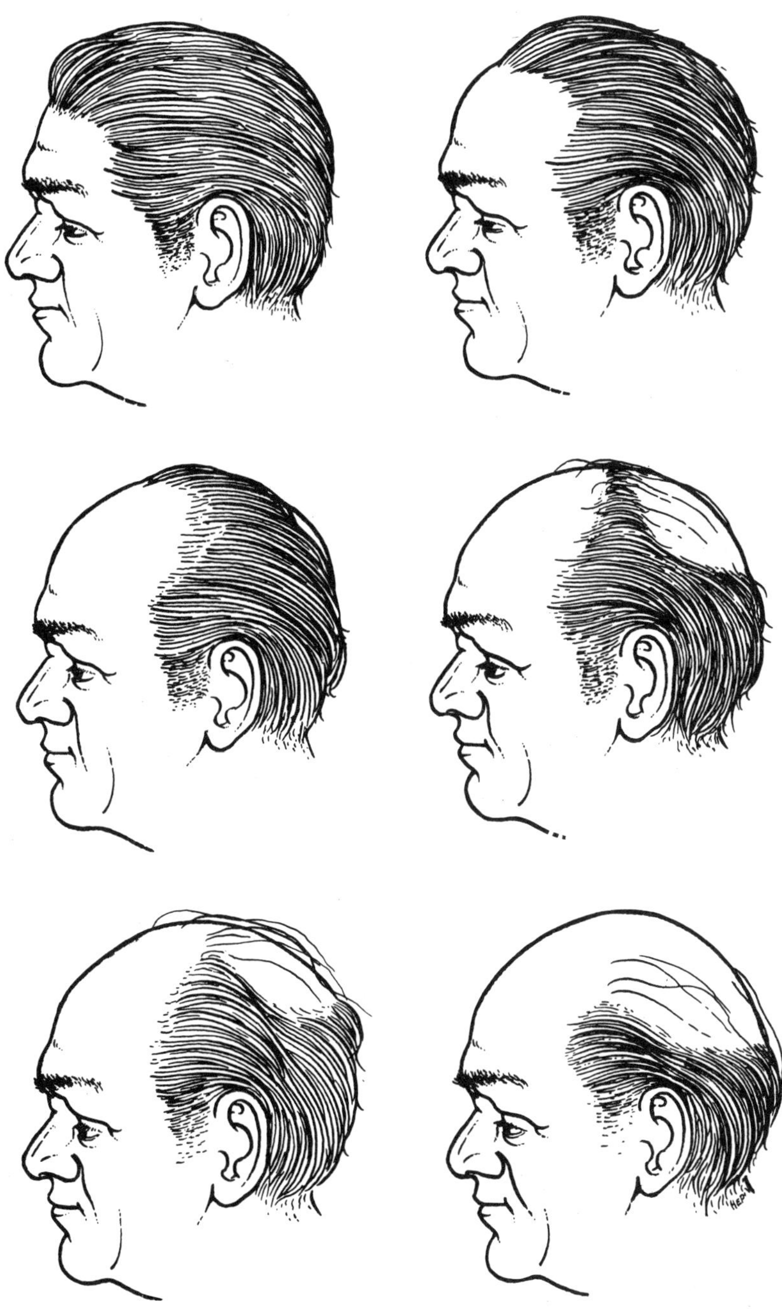

In 1959, Dr. Norman Orentreich, a New York dermatologist, first reported his technique of correcting certain cases of male-pattern baldness by use of hair plugs. Dr. Orentriech observed that grafts from the hair-bearing rim of the scalp were donor dominant, meaning they continued to grow even when transplanted into areas of baldness. Men who are even almost totally bald usually retain a rim of hair. Theoretically, the hair transplanted from this site would last the patient's lifetime if transplanted to the bald site. Unfortunately, we need more than just a thin rim.

Orentreich first described a technique of removing hair plugs, which contained fifteen to twenty hair shafts each, from the back and sides of the scalp, and then inserting them into the bald area. This procedure has been modified, but the principles remain basically the same.

The basis of the process of hair transplantation is that hair follicles from different parts of the scalp have what is called a "predetermined hereditary persistence potential," which remains even when hair is transplanted from one location to another. This is why areas of hair follicles with an expected longevity are those used in transplanting to the areas of hair loss. Because hairs from the lower occipital (back) and parietal (side) areas may be expected to persist more or less for a lifetime, it is these that are transplanted to the top areas of the male scalp, usually the area most prone to baldness.

Two different types of plugs can be used: the round plug, previously described, and a more recently developed square type. Other advanced techniques involve the use of a strip graft, a long hair-bearing strip of scalp tissue about fifteen centimeters long by eight to ten millimeters wide. These are commonly used in the frontal area, to give a new and more natural hairline. The strip graft avoids the cobblestone appearance that occurs when plugs are used on the anterior hairline. Finally, there are more surgically complex procedures that may give the best results available today for certain candidates. These involve the use of the so-called scalping flaps, which will be described later in this chapter.

Hair transplanted from one patient to another has not been feasible thus far. In certain experimental instances, hair so transplanted can survive when a steroid such as cortisone is injected into the grafted site. However, when the injections are stopped the hairs usually fall out.

CASE HISTORIES

John W., a thirty-six-year-old salesman, had been bald since the age of eighteen. He has lost the hair on the entire front and top area of his scalp, and was left with only a rather copious limb of hair in the parietal (side), occipital (back), and temporal (side) areas. John's father had a similar problem and eventually both were seen in consultation.

It was important to get a history of the parental pattern of balding. In this case, there was the advantage of my seeing the father, who, despite the fact that he was bald on the top of his head, had a fair amount of hair in the area most commonly used as the donor site. In his seventies, he had no need of correcting the balding pattern, and decided to accept the status quo.

However, John, who was looking for a new position, and who talked of starting a new business, was quite interested in hair transplantation. He had been adept at styling his hair and had allowed the hair at the temporal or side areas to get long enough so that he was able to comb it over the front of his head to cover some of the baldness. Nevertheless, this required a great deal of time each morning, more than he cared to spend, and despite all the styling, the look was still unnatural. John refused to wear a toupee so he came to me in the hope of obtaining a possible improvement. He was self-conscious and stressed that the result he wanted had to be natural in appearance. He had known other men who had had round and square hair-plug procedures, and was not particularly impressed with the results, especially in setting up the frontal hairline.

After thorough evaluation and discussion of the procedure, John elected to have the lateral scalp flaps performed in two stages. This involved taking a hair-bearing area from the side—or temporal—area of the scalp and relocating it by transplanting it to the frontal hairline, to establish hair up front that would then grow long and cover up, to a large degree, the balding area. The two stages of the procedure were separated by six weeks and done on an outpatient basis.

The technique involved the rotation of hair-bearing scalp from the temporal area without removal from the scalp. The flap is 12 centimeters long by 2.5 centimeters wide. This long and relatively narrow flap survives rotation and transplantation because of the good supply of blood that comes from the temporal artery, which is the blood source to the lateral area of the scalp. Both flaps, left and right sided, were turned anteriorly and then, in subsequent procedures, the patient had many hair plugs placed behind the flap to fill in this area further. One advantage of this flap method is that the normal density that existed on the side of the head is transplanted to the front area. The other is that there is not the usual fallout of hairs, as occurs in hair plugging, and so the result is immediate and far more satisfactory, although it involves more complex surgical techniques.

John W. found that the procedure achieved the natural results he had wanted, and that the hair transplantation helped him feel "more socially acceptable." His premature hair loss was the kind of limitation he felt compelled to change, and the rearrangement of his existing hairs achieved a desired goal. For him, the procedure was a success.

Another procedure was more satisfactory in its application with Marvin J., a twenty-eight-year-old school athletic instructor with a typical early balding pattern. Marvin was quite willing to undergo multiple procedures to correct as much of the problem as was realistic. But when I described the scalping flap process to him, he was not willing to undergo this type of surgery, preferring the hair plug procedure.

The process I used here encompassed five procedures, each involving a placement of about seventy-five plugs into the frontal and vertex areas of the scalp. The first seventy-five plugs were placed in the hairline, and all the subsequent plugs behind that initial hairline. Each of the procedures was done at approximately three-week intervals so that at the end of a three-month period, the basic 350 plugs had been placed. For this young man, the time spent and return visits were well worth it, and he was satisfied with the results.

Thomas Z., a fifty-four-year-old engineer, had a prominent widow's peak, which had been present for many years, and was now beginning slowly to extend. He had sparse hair throughout the rest of his scalp, and a desire to have his widow's peak "corrected." Although Thomas was not interested in a thick head of hair, he did want to have the anterior hairline corrected as much as possible.

Scalping Flap—Before and After

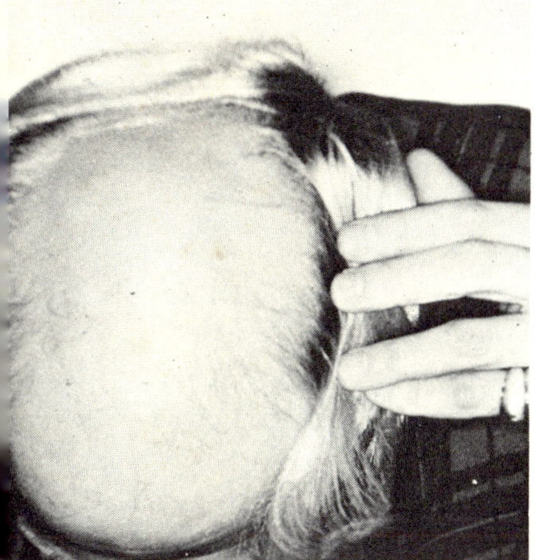

BEFORE

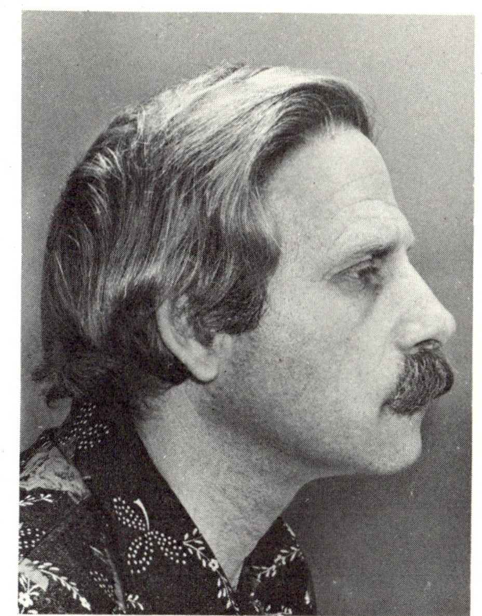

AFTER

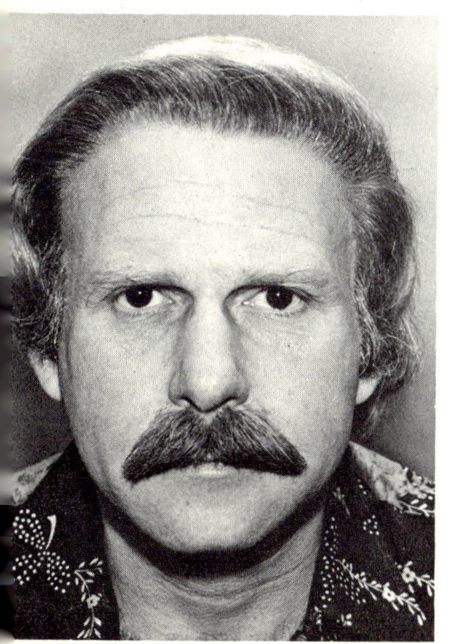

AFTER

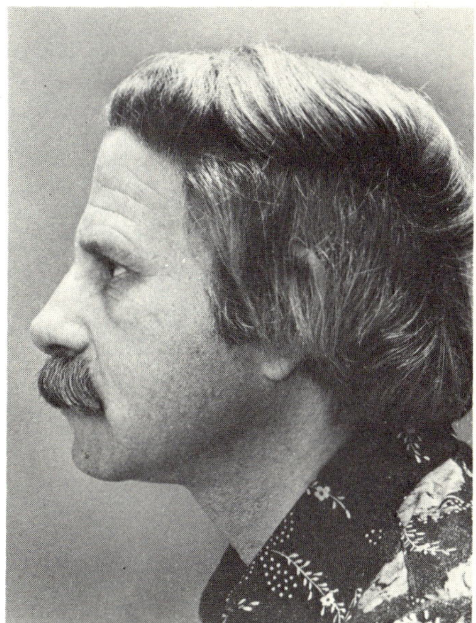

AFTER

In this situation, two procedures were done, each involving seventy plugs on each side, which corrected the hairline recession, made the widow's peak look less noticeable, and gave Thomas Z. an appearance that was much more satisfactory to his self-image.

SELF-EVALUATION

Obviously the test for baldness begins with your looking into the mirror and noticing that the normal position of the hairline is beginning to recede. Or, holding up a hand mirror, you may notice a vacancy becoming evident on the rear of your scalp. Or perhaps your wife or girlfriend has commented on a thinning area you haven't noticed. Suddenly you realize that the hairline you thought was only receding really has retreated or that spot of hair that was thin in back is so thin it's gone. With the sudden realization there can be trauma and the reality that you are losing your hair can be a

Strip Graft and Hair Plugs

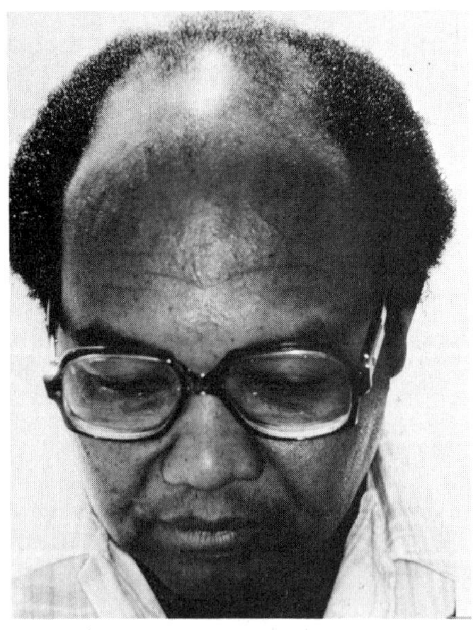

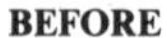

BEFORE

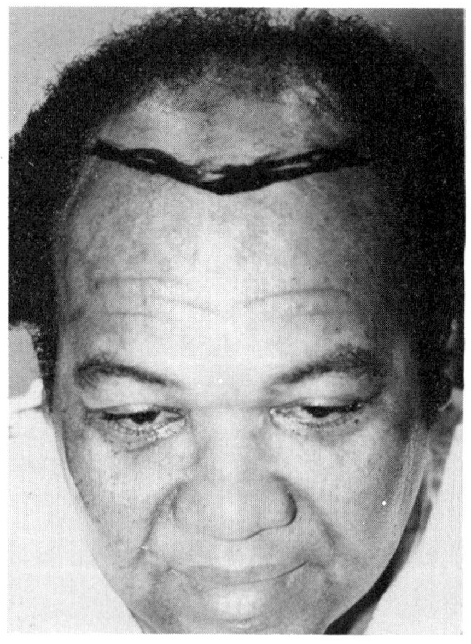

ALIGNING THE NEW HAIRLINE

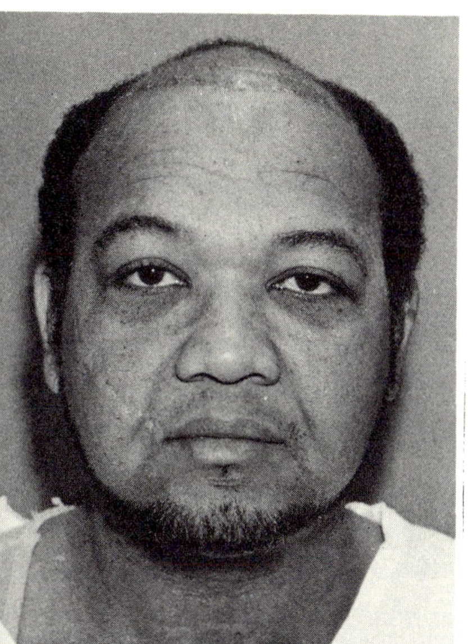

IMMEDIATELY AFTER

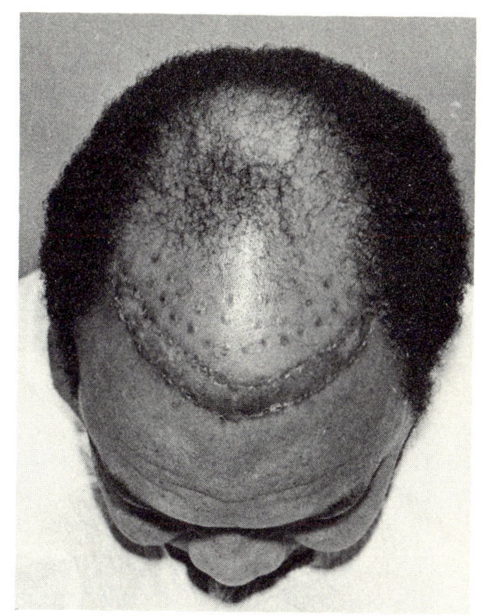

IMMEDIATELY AFTER

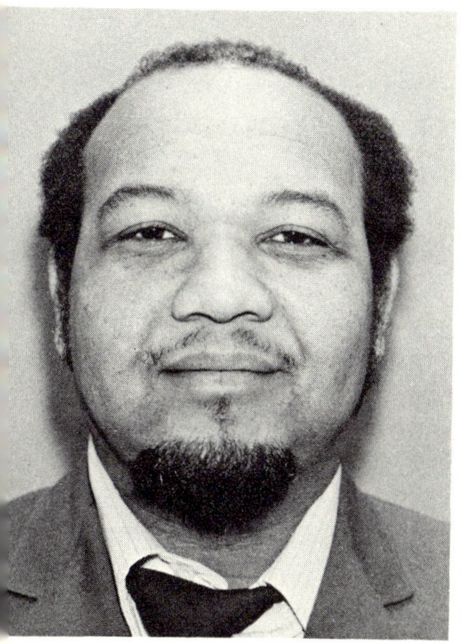

SIX MONTHS LATER

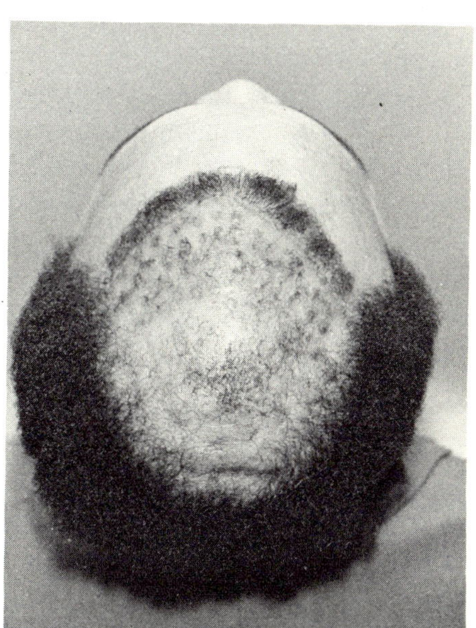

SIX MONTHS LATER
(Additional hair plugs needed)

forceful and frightening experience. Fortunately, you may be a candidate for hair transplantation.

There are a variety of male patterns of baldness, but when the process is complete, regardless of how it started, front or back, the result is frequently the familiar horseshoe-shaped fringe.

A surgical solution to replace hair loss is not for everyone. It demands patience, time, and an adequate amount of hair in the right places on the scalp to achieve a lasting and as natural an effect as possible. The results are far from instant and you should be aware of the commitment to be made and be realistic about the results that can be achieved. This is best discussed during your consultation with your surgeon.

We are born with a given number of hair follicles on the scalp and this endowment doesn't change. A full head of hair may have up to 100,000 hairs, and when hair transplantation is to be done, it is wise to realize that you can provide only your own source of hair, and therefore must have ample growth in the back and the sides of the scalp. We are only relocating the hairs that are present at the time of the transplant. If you don't understand this, then the costs, time, and benefits to be derived just might not be worth your efforts—and your surgeon's.

Incidentally, if you have any scalp condition, excessive dandruff or a scalp infection, you should first see a dermatologist and clear up the basic condition before considering any surgery. Your surgeon will advise you similarly and will likely ask you for a medical history as well.

BEFORE SURGERY

When a potential patient is inquiring about hair transplantation, I find it invaluable to discuss his medical history as well as any family history of balding patterns. It's important in any preoperative evaluation for a doctor to sit down with his patient and take the time to explain what the surgery can and cannot do.

One technique your physician may employ in this evaluation is to take photographs (which are frequently enlarged) so that the candidate becomes fully aware of all the dimensions of any problem areas by looking directly at them. It's amazing how few of us really understand how we look until a photograph is presented to us. I find this step often explains the magnitude of the problem to the patient in a dramatic way—one, in fact, which he may never have considered.

It's also important during this consultation to outline the level of the proposed new hairline. Most cases of baldness can be considerably improved by aligning, or setting up an anterior (front) hairline. In fact, one of the more common errors in doing this procedure, and which is frequently requested by the patient, is a hairline that would be too low and unnatural in appearance. It's difficult to create a low hairline: first, because it requires additional hairs that may not be available; and second, in a patient with a predictable balding pattern, it may lead to further hair fallout. Bald areas might occur behind the unrealistically low hairline, causing an unfavorable result.

Where there is a widow's peak, the problem can be corrected by hair plugs or strip-graft procedures. In more extensive cases of balding, the number of procedures that will more than likely be necessary should be explained to the patient by his doctor. These may include a combination of scalping flaps with hair plugs behind them, or the combination of strip grafts and square or round plugs also placed behind them. All these methods, including their pros and cons, should be discussed during your consultation so that you will have a complete understanding of just what can be done—including any and all limitations—and there will be no misunderstanding regarding expectation and actual outcome.

Hair transplantation does not usually require general anesthesia, but rather mild sedation, followed by a numbing solution of novocaine injected into the proposed operative site. You will probably be asked to be at the doctor's office or hospital about an hour before surgery, and given a mild sedative then. It can be supplemented by intravenous Valium during the procedure, if necessary. However, once the operative site is fully anesthetized, no further medications are usually necessary and no pain is experienced.

When it comes to the placement of the hairline it is important that both the patient and doctor agree, and for this reason I usually give the patient a mirror and a marking pencil. This is a wise precaution, one taken to avoid misinterpretation or misunderstanding later. The procedure will begin after both you and your surgeon agree on the placement of the hairline.

THE PROCEDURE

The hairs of the donor site, usually in the back or side of the head, are then clipped closely. Only the area that will serve as the source of the plugs is clipped so that the surrounding hairs are left long enough to cover the operative donor site. Your doctor will prepare the area to be repositioned by cutting the hair short, thus leaving stubble, rather than shaving off all the hair, so he can then observe the orientation of the hair follicles when they are procured; this is important from a technical point of view. Hair follicles come out at an oblique angle, rarely at 90 degrees. The punch (the instrument to procure the hair plugs) is then oriented along the direction of the hair shafts rather than at right angles so as to avoid any loss of critical hair follicles.

The area is usually prepped with standard iodine soap or pHiso-Hex soap solution. The proposed donor sites to be removed are outlined with a gentian violet marker to determine the number that will be procured so that an equal number of recipient sites can be punched out. When the anesthesia takes effect, usually after five minutes, the procedure begins.

One of the new technological advances that can help to minimize bleeding is the scalp hemostat, which is nothing more than an inflatable band that goes around the head. The pressure in the headband is increased by pumping a rubber bulb reaching a pressure of 150 to 250 millimeters of mercury. This decreases considerably the amount of bleeding and produces an almost bloodless field, which creates a clearer surgical site and substantially reduces the time necessary for the operative procedure. Because there is an absence of blood the patient's anxiety is also considerably reduced.

The plugs are removed by use of a hand-held biopsy punch, or with a motor-driven apparatus—a rotating cylinder that cores out the hair follicles. The number of punches that are taken during the procedure can vary from as few as twenty or thirty to up to as many as a hundred. Procedures involving more than a hundred plugs could be uncomfortable, and so if several hundred are necessary, the sessions should be extended over several periods of time, usually six weeks apart.

The hair-bearing plugs are placed into a sterile dish for later insertion into the recipient area, which has already been planned for

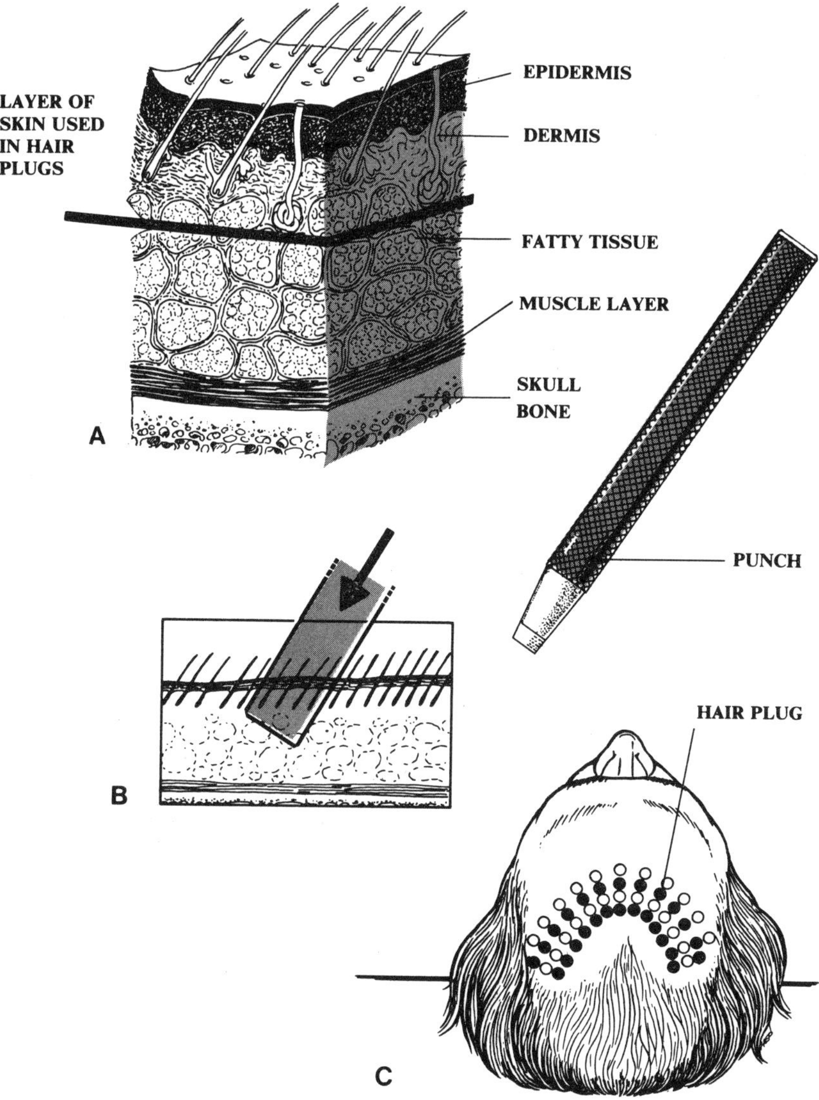

Plug Hair Transplant

A. *Cross section of the normal hair-bearing scalp illustrating the hair follicles and their relationship to the layers of the skin.*

B. *The hair punch used in the plug technique. It is placed in an angular direction to maximize the number of follicles to be obtained.*

C. *An example of the positioning of hair plugs. The white dots represent the first crop of plugs inserted. The darker dots represent subsequent placement of hair plugs.*

and outlined. The plugs are placed into punched-out sections in the balding area and are usually held there by pressure. The donor site is allowed to heal by itself, although sutures can be utilized to close it. Nevertheless, the site will heal and be nearly undetectable even if sutures are not employed. Overall, the utilization of sutures in the donor site minimizes the postoperative discomfort and allows for a faster-healing wound—and, theoretically, a slightly smaller scar. In the long run, however, the scarring is minimal. A light compression dressing of a non-sticking type is placed over the recipient and donor areas and the procedure is complete. The patient will be asked to return in a day or two to check the healing and to change the dressing.

Either strip-graft or scalping-flap techniques are also performed. In the strip-graft technique, the hair-bearing skin is taken from the posterior area and placed into a crescent-shaped recipient site that has been prepared for it in the anterior scalp. It will serve as the new anterior hairline. The donor site in the posterior area is usually closed by a running resorbable suture (which falls out or dissolves by itself). Closure of this wound is important to avoid extensive scarring in the area. When healed it is inconspicuous, and the resultant scar is covered by surrounding hair. The strip of hair-bearing skin is between four and six inches long and about half an inch wide. A number of hair plugs will subsequently be placed behind the new hairline; the number varies according to each individual case. The strip graft leaves a more natural hairline than plugs.

The scalping-flap procedure is a bit more elaborate. In this process, the hairs are not cut, but are left in their natural condition. There will be no fallout of hairs and subsequent regrowth, as in the

Opposite page: The Strip Transplant

A. The strip of hair-bearing scalp is removed from the back of the head.

B. A corresponding strip of the bald scalp is removed from the front of the head.

C. The hair-bearing strip is sutured into place.

D. Hair plugs are placed behind the strip graft to fill out the remaining bald area.

E. Several months later, the area is filling in.

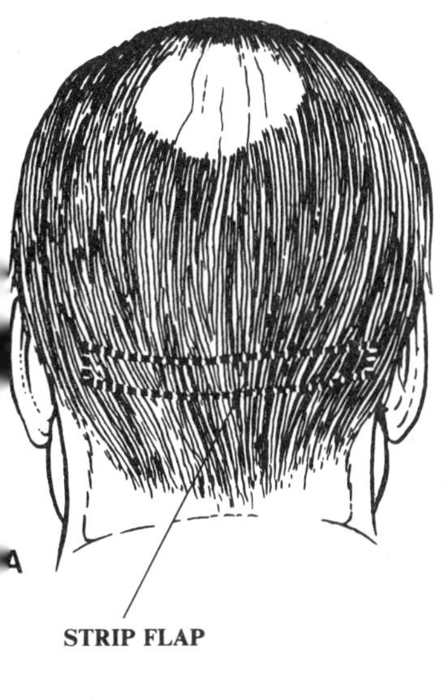
A
STRIP FLAP

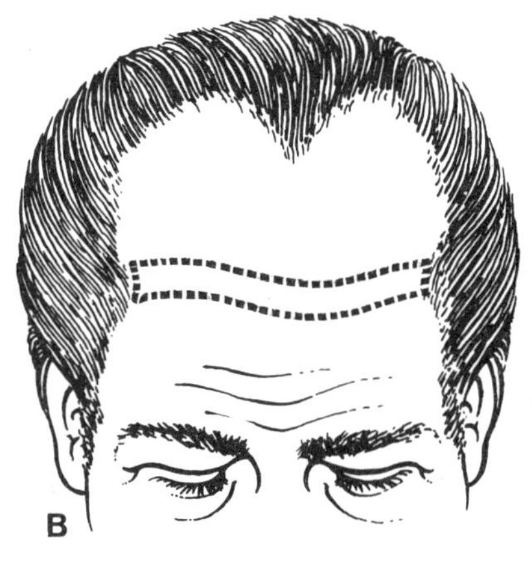
B

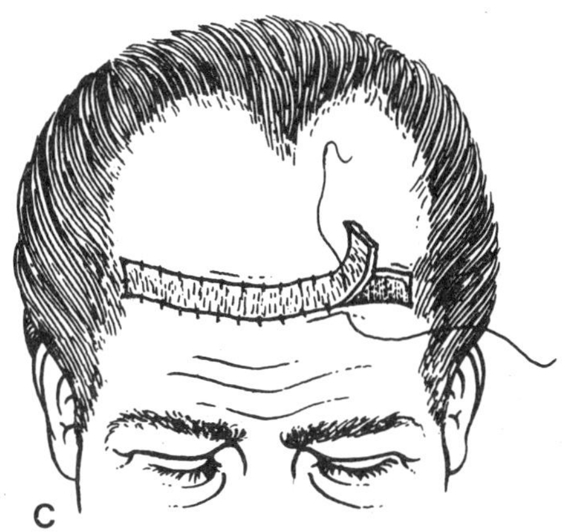
C

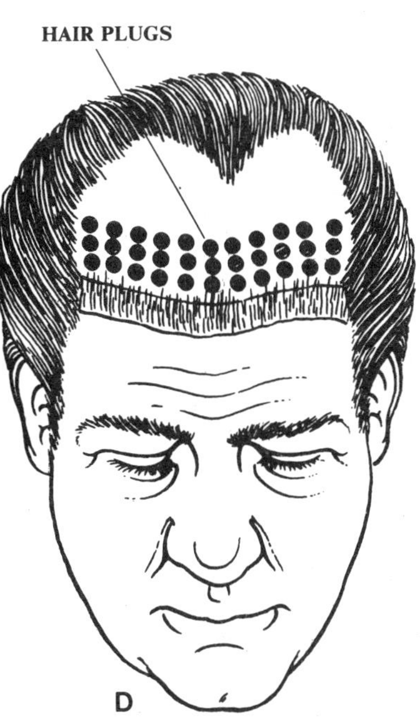
HAIR PLUGS
D

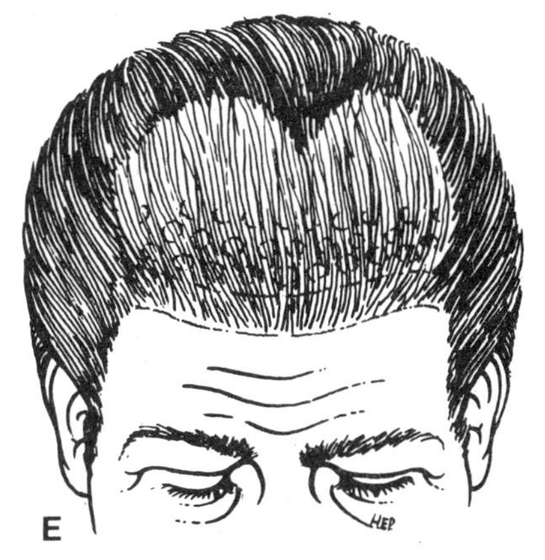
E

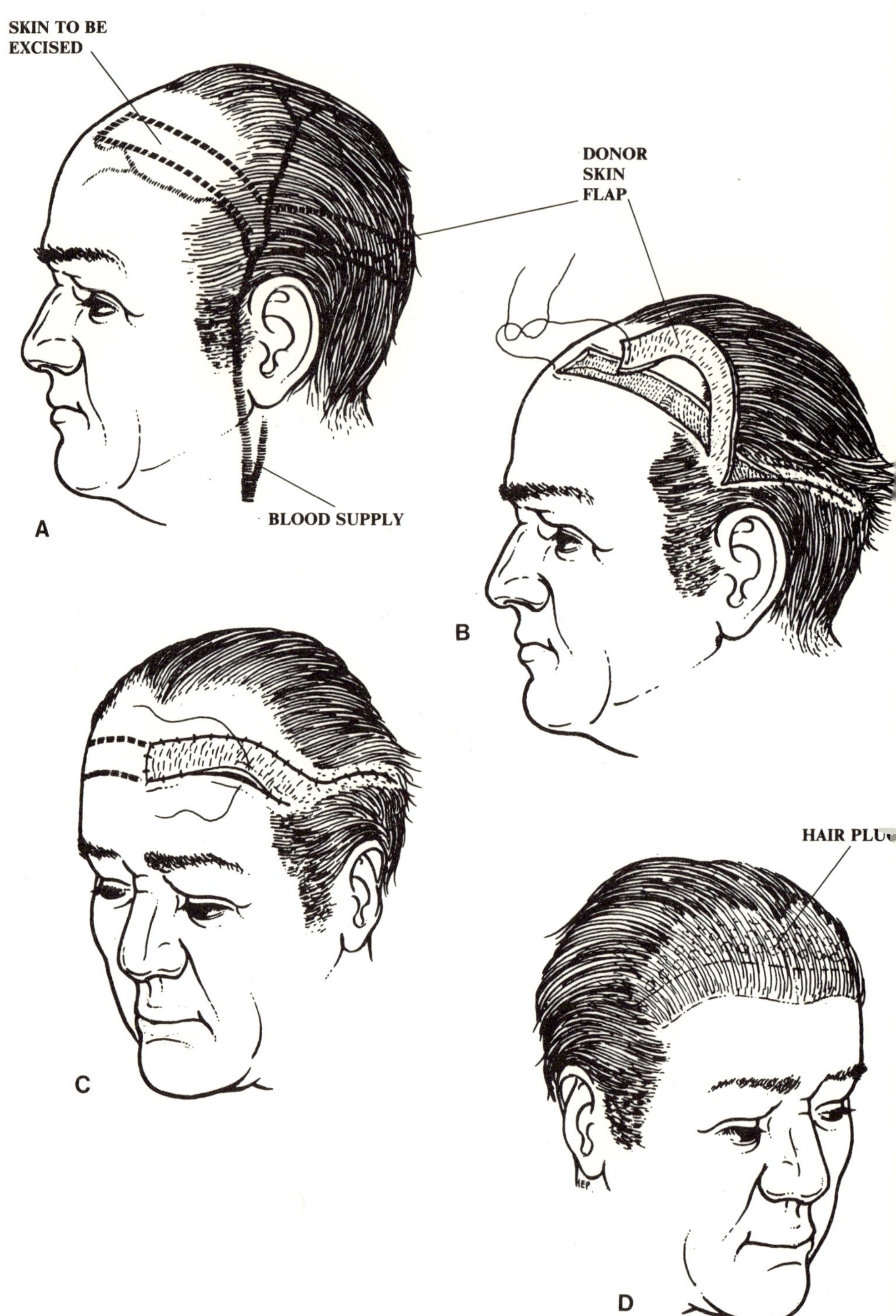
SKIN TO BE
EXCISED
DONOR
SKIN
FLAP
BLOOD SUPPLY
A
B
C
D

strip-graft or plug techniques. The scalping flap is outlined, elevated up, and rotated into position. It is inserted into an area in the anterior scalp. A one-inch by four- to six-inch section of non hair-bearing scalp is removed. A hair-bearing flap of the same size is sutured into its new position. The resultant defect in the side of the scalp is closed by bringing the edges together. This will result in a linear scar, which can be covered by the surrounding hairs. The scar is usually not hairline in thickness, though, because the defect that is closed is one inch wide. Closure under tension usually results in a sightly wide scar, although coverable by surrounding hair.

AFTER SURGERY

At the time of the first postoperative visit, any of the hair plugs that may have shifted beneath the dressing and are not aligned in their correct position can be reoriented, as there is still time to do so before they become firmly adhered to the scalp. Should this be necessary, it will take place within the twenty-four- to forty-eight-hour period during which you are asked to return. At this first postoperative visit the original dressings are removed and a lighter one applied. When the dressings are removed there may be some crusting around the plugs. This is due to oozing or seepage of tissue fluid. These crusts usually fall off within a week. You will be permitted to wash your hair and gently shampoo after the first few days.

Opposite page: The Flap Transplant

A. *A hair-bearing strip of the scalp, supplied by the temporal artery, is outlined on the side of the head. It is cut to lie in the front area, covering one-half of the front portion of the scalp.*

B. *The flap has been cut free except for a small attachment around which it is pivoted. The feeding artery is contained in this small scalp attachment. A corresponding strip of non-hair-bearing scalp is removed to receive the flap.*

C. *The flap is sutured into position. The area or donor site that it comes from is closed by pulling the scalp together with sutures.*

D. *The two flaps from the right and left sides have been turned into position, and hair plugs are placed behind them to further fill out the area.*

By skillful hair care, the recipient hair site and the donor site can be camouflaged with surrounding hairs. The plugs will contain short visible hair shafts that appear to grow, but will fall out. Subsequent new growth takes place in anywhere from three to four months later, but will be quite slow, and it will take eight to twelve months for the final length of the new hair transplant to occur. It is normal for the hair follicles to be in a state of shock as a result of transplantation. New hairs grow quite slowly—perhaps at the rate of half an inch a month, and this can be a distressing period. Eventually, there will be the growth you expected and a more natural appearance, but in hair transplantation, patience and time are vital factors.

It is important to realize that approximately two to three weeks after the intitial surgery all of the hairs will fall out—and that you should not think the operation has failed.

The percentage of hairs that "take" as a result of hair transplantation is approximately 98 to 100 percent if they are placed in nonscarred areas. Each of the plugs, approximately four or five millimeters in diameter, will contain twelve to sixteen hairs. A similar number of hairs should grow out in the next three- to six-month period.

WHAT CAN GO WRONG

Complications are rare, but should they occur, all are treatable. Infection will seldom occur, but can be treated with antibiotics and warm compresses if it does.

Another possible complication of the surgery could be bleeding. This is easily controlled by the placement of a suture at the time.

The technique involving the relocation of hair-bearing areas on the sides of the scalp (in the temporal area) that are then brought forward is a more complex procedure, and may create minor complications. The flap might not be placed perfectly in the hairline, or the most distal (distant) part of the flap may undergo some hair loss that may not be recoverable at the time of the initial surgery. The hair loss can be filled in at some later time with hair plugs, and if the hairline is not set adequately, minor revisions can be made later on.

• • •

WHAT YOU CAN EXPECT

Using any of the techniques I have described, and assuming that they are carried out with reasonable technical accuracy, you can expect a considerable improvement in your hairline and far greater density in the bald area than in the preoperative stage. However, it is impossible to regain the hair you once had before balding began, and it is very important for you to accept the basics of hair transplanting, namely that no new hairs are being placed into your head—we are merely rearranging or relocating what is already there. Assuming that the fallout rate stabilizes, and the hairs are successfully transplanted, they should stay and grow for a long period of time.

Many procedures are necessary to give a reasonably good result. These are often spaced over several weeks or months. The entire process—from beginning to end—in a massive hair loss case can take anywhere from six months to a year from the time of the initial surgery until you see truly satisfactory results.

In no other operation is patience so important, but no matter how patient you are prepared to be, you cannot and should not expect a full head of hair by any of the means now available to us in hair transplantation.

The use of the strip graft with hair-plug process will give you a considerable improvement. When feasible, the best results may be obtained with the scalping-flap technique—which gives a fairly natural hairline. Again, your expectations should be in proportion to your individual problem.

The expense of hair transplantation is usually not covered by insurance. The specific costs will vary with the methods used, and with just how many plugs are required in the punch-graft technique. Strip and flap procedures are generally more expensive, but—as previously mentioned—$10 per plug is a good approximation.

SIX

Blepharoplasty: The Eye-Lift Procedure

OUR EYES are our most expressive feature; they reveal a great deal about our emotions and our age.

The excess skin on the upper eyelid and the bagginess below signal the first signs of aging—a dissipated, spent look. It can occur even when we are young, get enough sleep, and generally take good care of ourselves, because some of us are born with a genetic predisposition to undereye pouches. These can affect our expressions and present an image to others that's different from the way we feel and see ourselves.

When chronically fatigued, our eyes reflect this condition; conversely, when rested, they have more sparkle. Bags under the eyes become more severe and the circles darken because of strain, insomnia, or anxiety. Bulging eyes may be the result of thyroid overactivity, and the heavy swollen look is occasionally associated with fluid retention in kidney diseases. Fortunately, most signs of aging around the eyes are just that—aging—and have no relation to general health.

The medical name for plastic surgery on the eyelids is blepharoplasty. It takes its root from the Greek words *blepharos,* which means eyelid, and *plastikos,* which means moldability. Thus, blepharoplasty literally means molding the eyelids.

Eyelid repair had its start not for cosmetic reasons, but because of visual problems. The early Arabs excised hanging skin from the eyelids when it impaired vision. While eyelid surgery actually goes back many centuries, it is only within the past two decades that major breakthroughs have occurred, resulting in an increase in the amount of such surgery being performed.

Cosmetic eyelid surgery took a giant step forward when in 1959 Dr. S. Castaneres described just how the periorbital fat that sur-

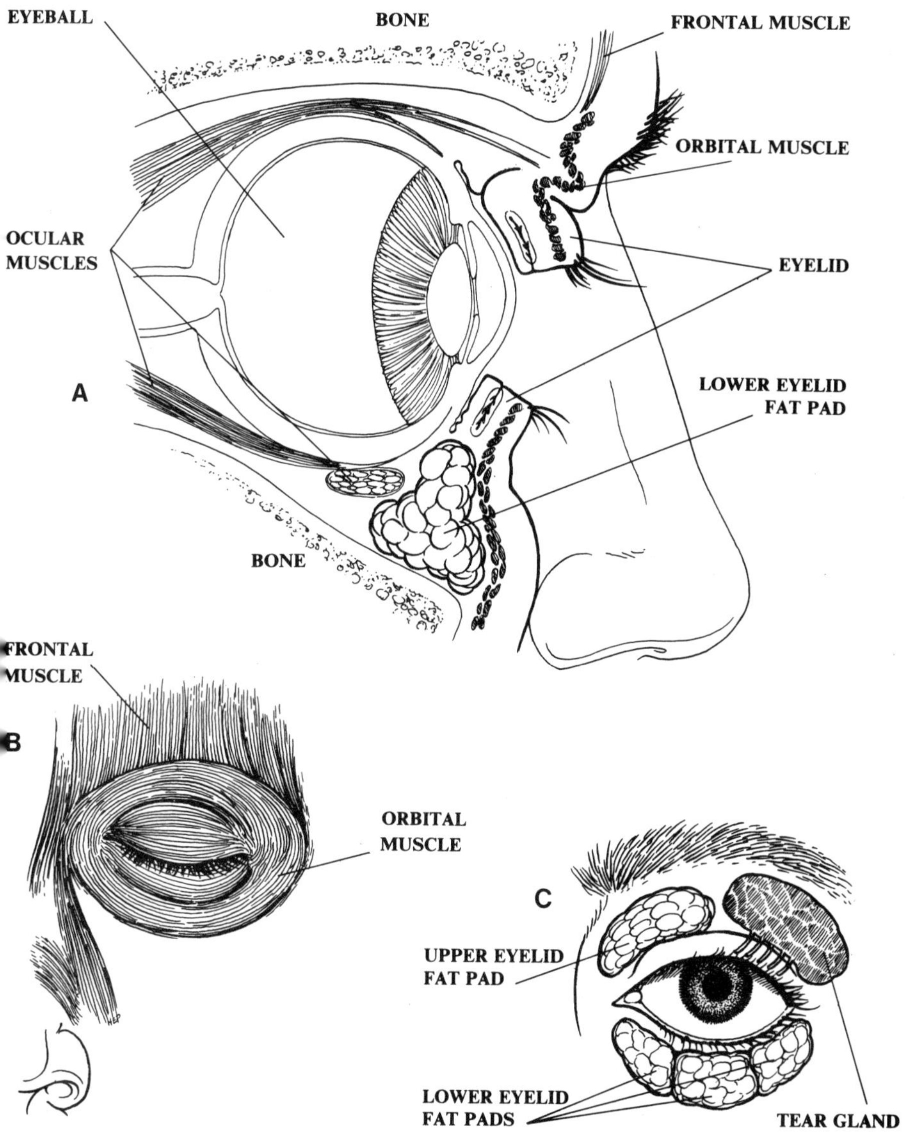

***Eyelid Surgery* (*Blepharoplasty*)**

A. *The anatomy of the eye, showing the eyelids and the fat of the lower lid area. Excess here causes bagginess.*

B. *The orbital muscle which encircles the upper and lower lid area.*

C. *The lacrimal, or tear, gland and the fat pad of the upper lid adjacent to the nose. This upper fat pad gives the fullness of the upper lid, resulting in the upper lid puffiness. The lower lid and its three distinct fat pad deposits are also shown.*

rounds the eye pushes through the retaining wall and results in puffy eyebags. There are three distinct fat pads in the lower eyelids, and when these fat pads push through the muscular retaining wall the result is pouchiness of the lower lids.

Another advance in plastic surgery involves the treatment of ptosis, or hanging in the lateral outer aspects of the eyebrow. Here, improved procedures have been developed to elevate and support the eyebrow in a more youthful position, so that a tired or so-called "hound dog" look can be eliminated.

Most recently, a procedure has been perfected that allows for a better alignment of the upper-eyelid fold, maintaining a younger look. As for the lower eyelid, techniques have now been developed that permit the removal of moderate amounts of skin, while avoiding the pulling down of the lower eyelid—a condition called ectropion.

These developments and improved techniques within the past three decades have enabled today's plastic surgeons to accomplish subtle and dramatic eyelid improvements that help eliminate a tired, older appearance.

CASE HISTORIES

Most men who come to the office complain that they look "too old" or "too tired," and inquire about a face-lift. When we discuss the possible results of the face-lift procedure, the conversation almost invariably turns to those bags and pouches under the eyes. I often suggest combining face and eye surgery to many of my patients, and an increasing number of men as well as women are now having the face-lift and eye-lift procedures done simultaneously.

One such patient is Jim F., a tennis pro from Long Island, New York. Jim's fifty-one years old and in terrific shape. When he came to see me, he knew beforehand that he wanted both a face-lift and eye surgery—the face-lift to get rid of wrinkles and the eye-lift to eliminate not only bags under his eyes but also extra skin in his upper lids. The upper-lid condition was obviously inherited, because Jim's eighty-five-year-old mother had so much extra tissue in this same area that it was literally obstructing her vision. (By the way, keep in mind that if an operation is performed because of vi-

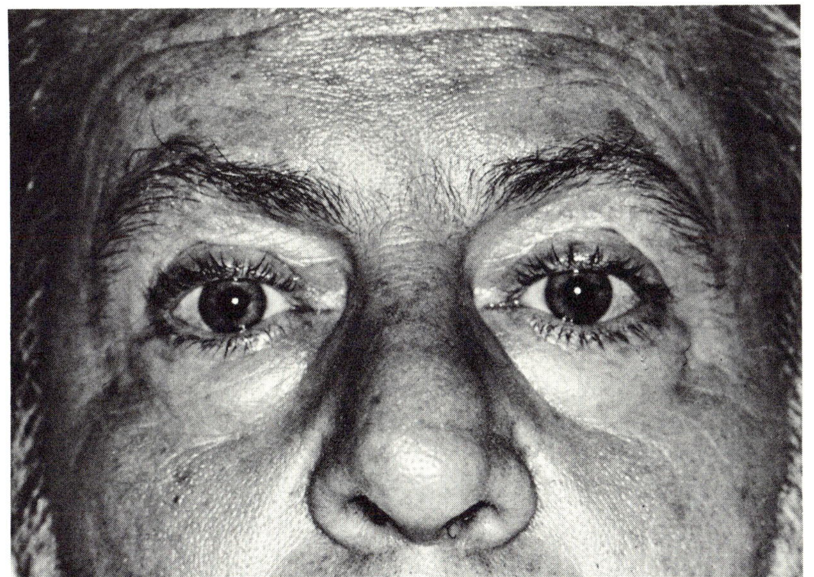

BEFORE

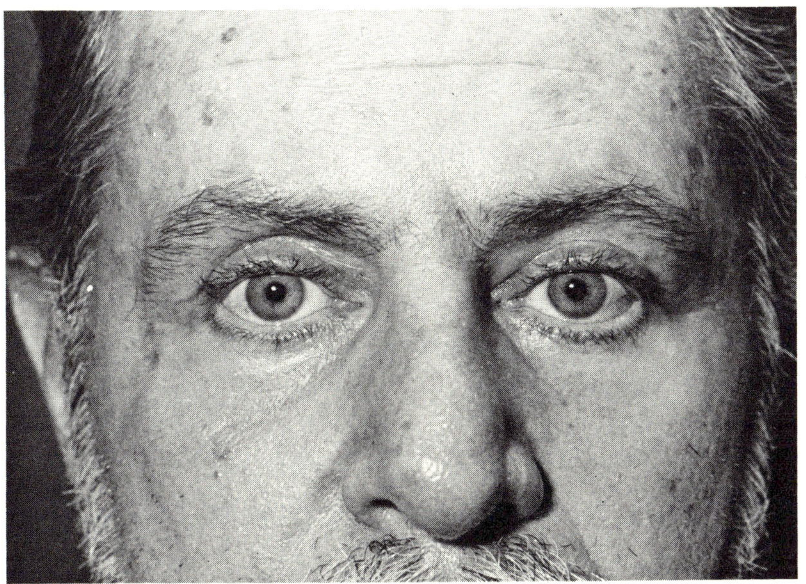

AFTER

Eyelid Surgery (Upper and Lower Lid)—Before and After

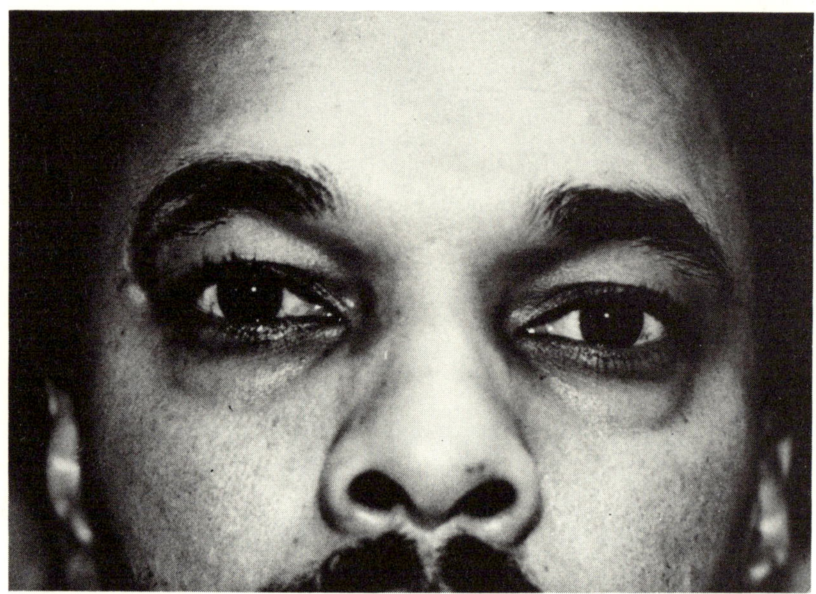

BEFORE

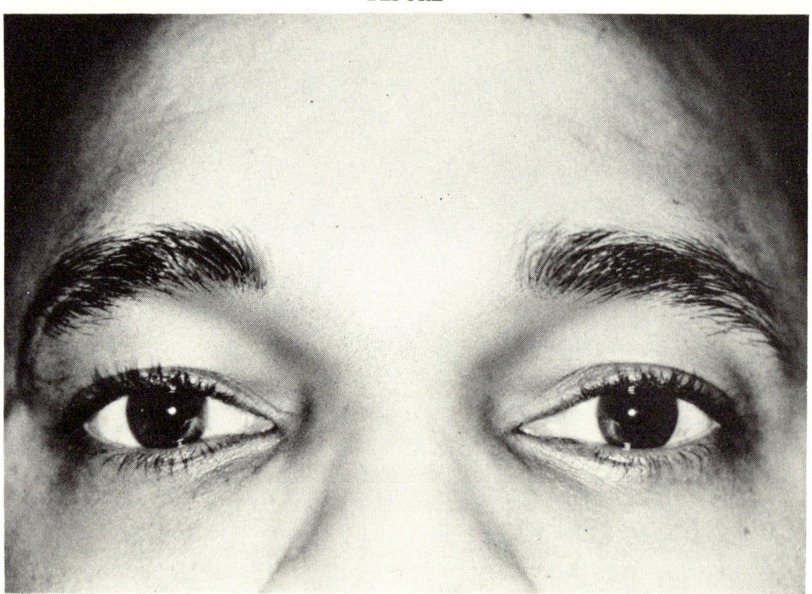

AFTER

Eyelid Surgery (Lower Lid Only)—Before and After

sion impairment, and it is documented by an ophthalmologist, it may very well be at least partially covered by insurance.) In Jim's case, I performed both procedures on the same day, and both were equally successful.

Ken F., a tall, attractive man, was thirty-four years old when we first met. He was in good health, had an equally attractive wife and two small children, and a job with an international electrical equipment manufacturer. Ken was in the financial department and had hopes of one day becoming controller of the company.

According to Ken, there was a stumbling block in the way of corporate advancement. He was hearing phrases like "Wow, what a night you must have had!" This was because of the bags he carried under his eyes—bags, by the way, that he had carried since his teens. Lately this kind of remark had been coming from executives of other divisions within the company. Ken, who was insecure about his position there, was concerned that he would be thought to be burning both ends of the candle, when, in fact, he was a hard working, sober individual who went to bed early every night.

Ken never liked the look of his eyelids, but was now even more concerned that an undeserved appearance of debauchery could ruin his chances of climbing up the corporate ladder. He came to see me about what might be done to improve his appearance.

Although Ken was young, the pouchiness made him look much older and more tired than he was. The heavy undereye bags spoiled an otherwise handsome face, and after discussion, we both decided that Ken could benefit from removal of the pouches around the lower lids as well as some sagging of the upper eyelids. The procedure was a success. Today the tired look is gone and so are the pouches, while Ken feels much better about himself and his chances in his company.

Usually I do the upper and lower eyelids together; most men usually need both corrected. If there is puffiness and bagginess in the lower area, chances are there is also extra skin in the upper portion. Most men who are concerned about their eyes stress the lower lids as the problem area; after consultation they often realize that the elimination of extra skin on the upper lid will also be needed to give a more youthful appearance.

A forty-three-year-old man, Steven B., recently divorced, wanted to enter the single social scene again. He came to me to get rid of the "tired" look around his eyes. An operation took care of the extra skin in the upper part of the eyelid and excessive puffiness in the lower, and Steve is quite satisfied with the results.

A well-known lawyer, William M., recently inquired about eye surgery for himself after he saw how well his wife looked after similar surgery. William, a huge, tall man with a beard, was concerned that his eyes, which were dramatic and more obvious since he wore a beard, gave him a tired look. I operated and effectively got rid of that problem for him.

SELF-EVALUATION

Look in the mirror, take a pinch of the skin of your upper eyelid—that area between the eyebrow and the upper eyelash. Do you think you look better now? If so, then more than likely you're a candidate for a blepharoplasty.

If you want to test yourself as to whether or not your lower lids are too puffy, first close one eye and then gently push on that upper eyelid. If you observe with your other eye a bulge or the pushing-out of fat, then fat-bag excision might be considered.

When you have a ptotic—drooping—brow, you more than likely can see it as it is. If you still want to test yourself, put a finger on your eyebrow and see how it lies in relation to the bone over the eye—the orbital ridge. This sharp-edged bone represents the upper-outer portion of the eye socket. If your eyebrow is at the same level or above the orbital rim, ptosis probably is not a problem. But if the eyebrow hangs below the ridge, then corrective surgery can elevate it and also minimize the amount of excess skin in the upper lid.

I always point out to prospective patients that there are many factors affecting the eyes and how they appear. For instance, some eyes look worse in the morning, but as the day wears on the pouch bags beneath become less obvious. The effects of gravity have much to do with this. When you awake in the morning there is a puffy look, but after you have been upright for several hours, these pouches will become less apparent, although they may never completely disappear.

A medical checkup is advisable shortly before any cosmetic surgery, particularly eyelid surgery. This is especially so for the older patient. Certain diseases and medical conditions can affect the eyelids and require a doctor's approval before the procedure can begin. A long-standing hyperthyroid condition, for example, can cause thickening of the eyelid skin, creating droopiness and bagginess, and a frequent stary or "bug-eyed" look. The tissue surrounding the eye swells, pushing the eyeball out. It is important that a person with this ailment get back to a normal thyroid balance before the plastic surgery is performed. Similarly, a person with a malfunctioning kidney or heart may accumulate fluid in the eyelid area; certainly these conditions should be controlled before blepharoplasty is contemplated.

I have also encountered patients who have been on a long-term steroid treatment for any one of a variety of diseases. These individuals tend to have a tremendous amount of edema, or swelling, around the eyelid area. This condition also should be taken into account before surgery is decided upon.

Allergic conditions also should be brought under control, for they can cause a great deal of swelling about the eye area—as do conditions that bring about spasms of blinking.

There are, as you can see, certain medical and ophthalmological conditions that can put off or even preclude eye-lift surgery. These are usually rare, and in most cases men of any age can get medical approval for the surgery.

BEFORE SURGERY

During consultation with your surgeon he will test the tissue laxity and bagginess surrounding your eye, and will give you his expert opinion on the amount of improvement you can expect. More often than not, as we have already discussed, fat bags around your lower and upper eyelids can be removed and excess skin of your upper eyelid trimmed. It is important, however, that sufficient skin remain for the eyelid to close easily. Surgery should not cause any impairment of your vision. As a matter of fact, if your upper eyelid creates a hooded effect, the skin removed may even improve the range of your upper and lateral visual fields. If you're looking a bit saggy or baggy around your eyes then more than likely blepharoplasty can help.

Here are some of the more common eyelid complaints and a brief description of how surgery can be effective in taking care of them.

Suppose you have extra upper and lower eyelid skin. In such a case, the simple elliptical excision of skin in the upper and lower eyelid area should be effective. How much loose skin you have may be a matter of subjective opinion; obviously if the skin is obscuring vision, it's the right time for surgery. Or if a less dramatic amount of excess skin is esthetically offensive to you, you may also be ready.

No matter what your age, if you have fat that is herniated or bulging, causing bagginess, you may want to have eye-lift surgery. The appearance of your eyelids will benefit from the removal of the excess fat. In the lower-lid area, little or no skin has to be removed unless there is an excess of it, and then only a millimeter or so. This avoids the undesired pulled-down look of the lower lid.

Perhaps you have a longitudinal roll of tissue just beneath the eyelid margin that gives a thickened appearance to the lower eyelid. This thickened appearance is caused by an actual thickening or hypertrophy of the orbicularis muscle, the muscle that controls the opening and closing of the eyelid. This can be corrected in surgery by a partial resectioning of the muscle. (Note that the orbicularis is not one of the muscles responsible for eyeball movement. They are never touched.)

If you're sporting a few more crow's feet—those very fine lines that are sometimes referred to as "laugh lines"—and they extend into the lateral or outer aspect of the eyelid area and onto the cheeks, excision of the skin probably won't be adequate to remove them. Blepharoplasty will not eliminate horizontal lines around the eyes, or excessively wrinkled skin around the area to be operated on. Other procedures, such as chemical peeling, can improve the situation and may have to be employed as a secondary procedure.

When your brow is ptotic, or droopy, particularly in the upper-outer aspect, the simple excision of tissue from the eyelid area will not be the solution. In fact, excision of excessive eyelid skin brings the brow farther down and can accentuate the problem. There are other procedures that can correct the condition, such as a transverse elliptical excision of tissues above the brow, farther up in the forehead, or in the scalp in an area covered by hair.

These are some of the more familiar problems involving the areas around the eyes. They are not the only ones. You may have another condition that you want to discuss with your plastic surgeon. Depending on his age, his complexion, and the results of an inherited condition, each individual has special needs and requirements, and therefore no single surgical technique is tailor made for everyone. That is why consultation and discussion are important for you and your doctor. Your surgeon should be receptive and thorough and tell you as precisely as he can what results he may achieve for you. And you should feel comfortable in expressing all your feelings about the subject too.

The technical aspects of blepharoplasty are not complicated, but demand extreme precision and control; millimeters count on the eyelids. The procedure can be performed in a hospital or at a doctor's-office operating room. It is usually done with local anesthesia.

The night before the operation you will be asked to wash your face thoroughly with an antibacterial soap. The next day, before being taken to the surgery area, you will be given mild sedation with a hypodermic needle. In the operating room, some intravenous Valium will be administered for further sedation. Sedatives are given sparingly because your surgeon will need your cooperation during the procedure, but be assured that you will be given enough to alleviate all anxieties.

To outline the incisions to be made, the doctor will use his forceps to pick up the amount of skin to be excised from the upper eyelid and outline it with a marking pen. He will then outline the incision to be made in the lower eyelid area in a similar manner.

A very fine hypodermic needle is used to inject a novocaine solution containing epinephrine (also called adrenalin) into the skin of the eyelid area. This numbs the lid and also allows for the shrinkage or constricture of blood vessels. Some slight discomfort might be felt, but it only lasts a few seconds, and after it is done you will feel no pain. An antibiotic ointment will also be applied to your eyes in order to protect them, which will blur your vision temporarily.

THE PROCEDURE

Once the anesthesia has taken effect the surgeon will excise a strip of skin from the upper eyelid. He probably will also excise a strip of muscle so that he can see the orbital fat protrude through the incision in the upper eyelid. The fat pads are then removed. The removal of any fat from the upper eyelid may cause some slight discomfort and a feeling of pressure. This rapidly disappears after the fat is removed.

The surgeon now goes to the lower lid—an area that is a bit more critical to work with because there tends to be less skin available for removal. Here judgment is critical. An incision is made approximately one millimeter below the eyelash. The skin is lifted away and another incision is made through the muscle of the lower eyelid, allowing the fat bags to become visible. By placing a slight pressure on the upper eyelid, the three localized fat bags in the lower-lid area can be correctly determined and identified. During the fat removal procedure an electrocautery needle may be used to coagulate any of the blood vessels that might tend to ooze postoperatively.

When the fat has been removed the physician will determine the amount of skin that can be excised. He will probably ask you to open your mouth wide and to look all the way up to the ceiling so that he can better judge how much skin to remove. This is important, for if too much is taken away, ectropion (the lower eyelid pulled down) can develop.

The entire blepharoplasty procedure takes an hour or less from start to finish. When the operation is over, cold compresses will be applied to the eyes or an occlusive eyepatch dressing will be used for a few hours. For those patients who suffer claustrophobia from having their eyes closed, I assure them that they can remove the dressing if necessary. The simple knowledge that the patches can be

Opposite page: Eyelid Surgery (Blepharoplasty)

A. *Excision of the skin above the eyebrow for a brow lift, and excision of the upper eyelid skin.*

B. *Removal of skin and closure of the wound. The dotted line shows the incision site for lower lid surgery. Notice that it is immediately below the lower eye lashes, so that when it has healed, the incision is nearly invisible.*

C. *Removal of the lower lid fat pads: the skin is elevated, and finger pressure reveals the bulging fat pads. Excess skin is removed and the new skin edges are sutured together.*

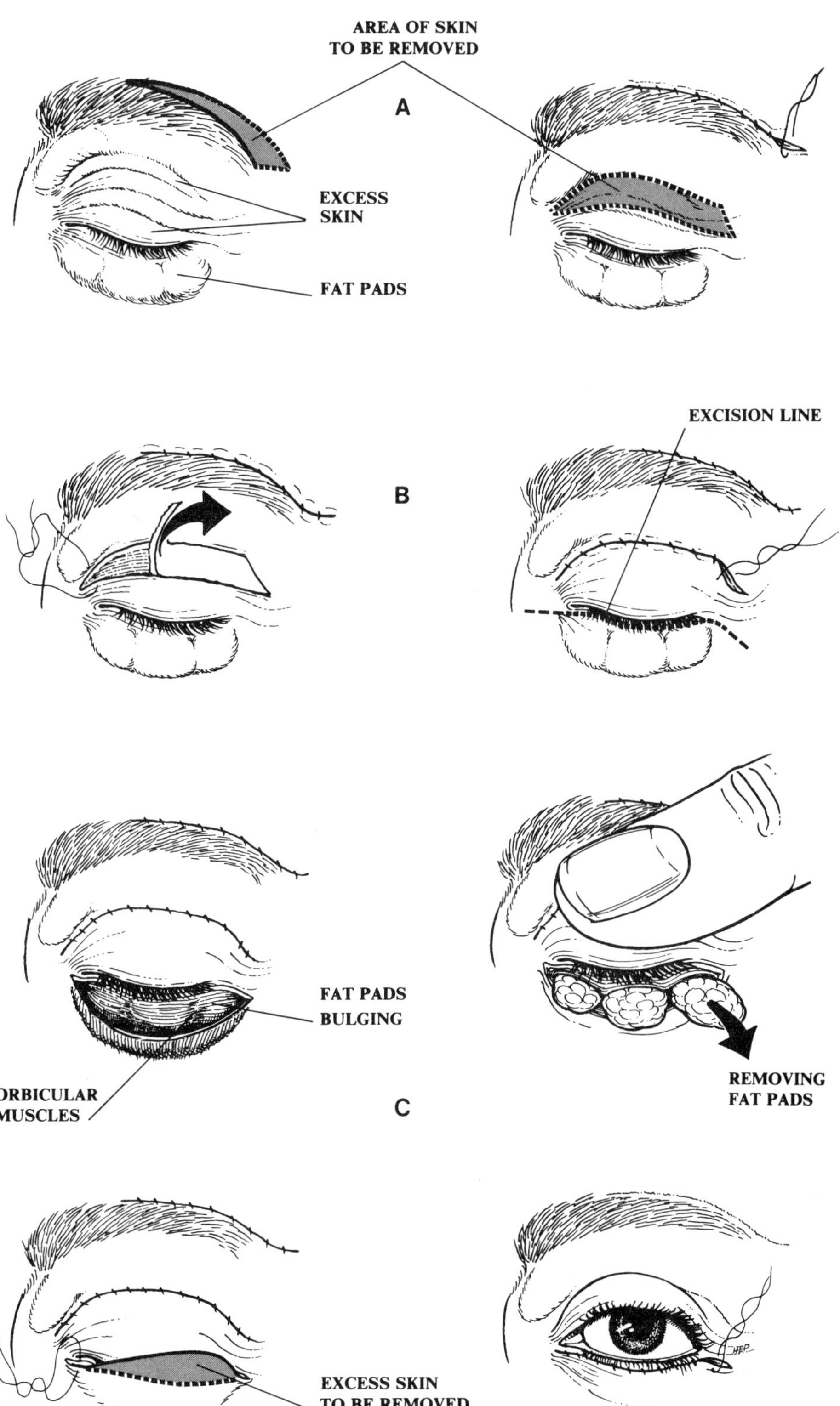
AREA OF SKIN
TO BE REMOVED
A
EXCESS
SKIN
FAT PADS
B
EXCISION LINE
FAT PADS
BULGING
ORBICULAR
MUSCLES
C
REMOVING
FAT PADS
EXCESS SKIN
TO BE REMOVED

taken off is usually enough to sustain the patient to wear them for just an hour or two. You don't have to be blindfolded.

AFTER SURGERY

Immediately after the operation your head will be elevated and the nurse in attendance will apply cold compresses to reduce the swelling and bruising. Sutures are removed on the fourth or fifth day after surgery. By the tenth day, the telltale signs, any swelling and bruising, will have subsided or be nearly resolved. Final resolution takes a few more weeks.

You will be astonished to learn how unobservant most people are. You needn't worry too much about non-family members noticing your eyelid change. Very few are that keenly aware. They may see you in toto, but rarely will they scrutinize you in detail. A more relaxed, alert look is all that will be apparent to anyone looking at your eyes. Weeks after, your friends may comment on how well you look.

You may want to wear sunglasses in public to conceal any redness at the incision sites, or the minimal bruising that still may be evident after seven to ten days. After removing your glasses, if you want to keep your operation secret when you begin to receive compliments, you might casually mention how you've been upping your sleep quota of late, and that it has been a life saver. Then again, if you want to be honest, why not share your eye-lift experience with interested friends? After all, it is getting to be a commonplace procedure, and there is certainly nothing to be ashamed of for having improved your appearance.

WHAT CAN GO WRONG

A variety of annoying situations can occur, none serious and all correctible. One problem that crops up is the brow hanging below its proper level. When the upper lid is operated on, the removal of skin can cause the brow to sag even more. So in addition to taking out a strip of skin to create a nice youthful fold, it may be advisable to perform a brow-lift or a forehead procedure.

Ectropion, however, can be a temporary result of postoperative swelling, and in this case the condition will go away when the swelling goes down. You may have to tape the lower lid so that it lies firmly against the eye until the swelling decreases.

A situation may occur when not enough fat is removed from the eyelids, particularly the lower lid area. This can easily be corrected by a minor secondary procedure. The surgeon, however, will be careful not to remove too much fat; otherwise the eyes will take on a sunken apearance. Proper judgment on the part of the surgeon is essential—when to excise enough fat to remove the baggy look, but when to stop removing it so that a hollow-eyed look doesn't develop.

It you are contemplating blepharoplasty you may feel safe in assuming that blindness will not result from the operation. There have been rare cases where a patient has become blind in one eye after the operation, but no causal relationships have been found. A variety of other situations are thought to have been responsible—preexisting medical conditions such as glaucoma, diabetes, multiple sclerosis, and brain tumors or aneurisms.

Overall, most problems of the blepharoplasty are temporary and disappear soon after the operation. Eyelid repair is one of the safest procedures performed, and one that can give a dramatic improvement to your appearance.

WHAT YOU CAN EXPECT

It's two to three weeks after surgery. The reflection in the mirror pleases you. You're studying yourself as you shave and you look closely at the work that has been done on your eyes. The scars in the normal crease of the upper eyelid and right under the lash line in the lower lid are already definitely less visible. Your eyes will appear larger and more wide open. Any drowsiness or sleepiness in your facial expression—that dim quality—is gone.

If you are in your forties, and upper-lid treatment is all you needed, you'll be elated about your new youthfulness. If your problem was under-eye bags becoming more prominent (occurring more often in the late forties or fifties, unless it is a condition that you were born with and that has worsened with age), the smooth expanse of skin from your cheeks to your lashes may seem almost miraculous to you. You will look more refreshed and enjoy the benefits that go with it.

SEVEN

Otoplasty: Ear Surgery

QUICK. Don't look. Now try and describe your ears. Difficult? No, you're not unobservant. Few of us can clearly describe what our ears look like because there is really little that is noteworthy or distinguished about the human ear, unless, of course, it is partially absent or deformed. And yet, at the same time, the elevations and contours of the ear—its component parts—are rather difficult to reconstruct.

Try pinching yourself. First on your face, then behind your ear. You can feel that the area behind the ear is relatively insensitive. It's why cosmetic surgery on this area is just about the easiest and most painless kind of surgery to perform. The operation is delicate but uncomplicated, because there are no bones to break, no masses of skin that have to be undermined, and no large areas that require lengthy incisions.

The ear is actually divided into three distinct parts: the outer, middle, and inner. As a plastic surgeon, my concern is with the outer—the visible—ear. Let's take a brief look at it.

The outer ear is first formed from six distinct elevations in the five-week-old embryo, and then rapidly progresses to the final adult shape. By the time one is born the ear is fully formed. The function of the outer ear is both to protect the middle and inner ear and provide a conduit through which sound waves enter the auditory canal. It consists of a shell of cartilage that is covered with skin; almost no fat is between this skin and cartilage, and so our ears are highly sensitive to any changes in temperature.

The ears attain full development by the time we're four or five years old. It takes the rest of the body years to catch up, so that a child's ears may seem disproportionally large. And, if they also protrude, the awkwardness will be even more apparent. It was once

EMBRYOLOGY

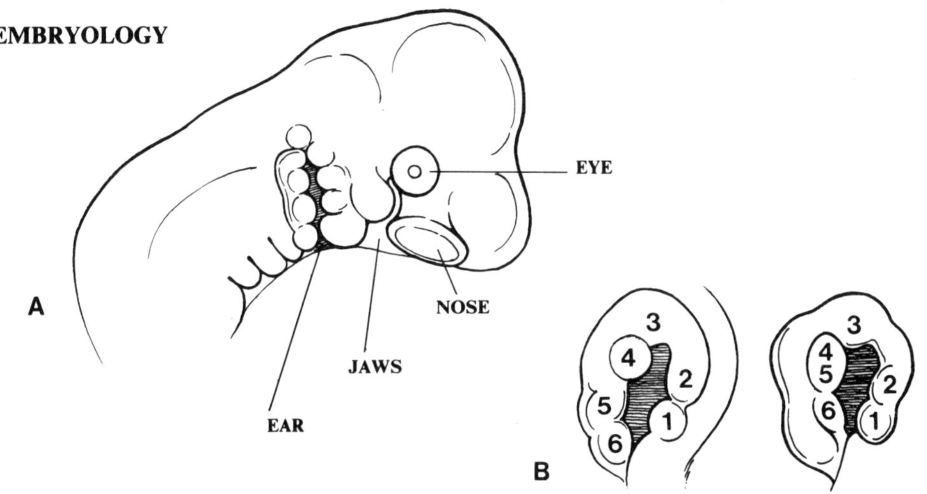

ANATOMY

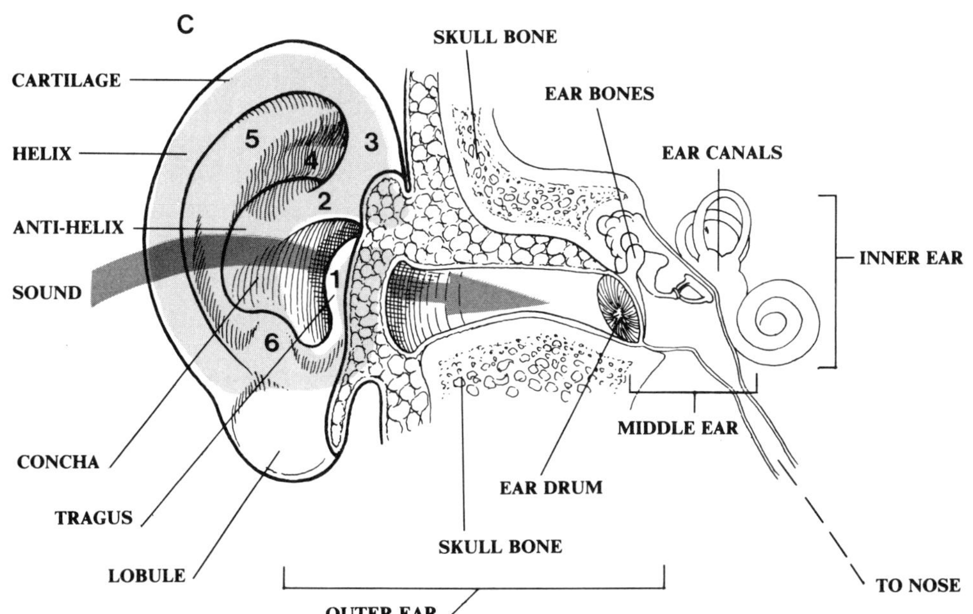

The Embryology and Anatomy of the Ear

A. The embryo at a few weeks reveals the location of the future facial parts.

B. A close-up view of the developing external ear. The distinct parts of the adult ear have developed from vague embryologic elevations.

C. The outer, middle, and inner ear anatomy. The external ear parts are derived from the embryonic folds or elevations seen in A.

thought that there is a growth spurt of the ear as we get older. Not so. What happens is that as we mature our features begin to shrink and everything starts to sag. The ears, however, don't—except, perhaps, for the lobules—because the cartilage structure usually stays and keeps the ears firm. And so, as we age, the ears may appear to get bigger.

What is truly remarkable about the human ear is how much it differs on each individual; its shape and size, like fingerprints, are unique. Different ethnic groups and races also have differing types of ears. The Japanese, for instance, have lobes that are connected by skin to the upper region of the neck. In some individuals, vestigial muscles surrounding the ear can still be used to wiggle it. The skin behind it, which closely matches facial skin, is often employed in skin grafting.

Since the ear is so different from one individual to another, and indeed, from one side of the head to the other, it would be unrealistic to expect a plastic surgeon working on one ear to produce a mirror image of the other. However, while all ears are different, most men don't want their ears to be *too* different.

The culture and mores of a society can also be a factor. England's Prince Charles is rumored to have had corrective surgery on ears that once seemed to protrude noticeably, but which do not appear to do so in current photographs. A Japanese man, on the other hand, probably wouldn't have similar cosmetic surgery, because large ears are a sign of good luck in Japan. Men can be dissatisfied if their ears protrude too much, are too cupped, too shell-like, or too pointy.

I often meet patients who have come to me for a consultation about cosmetic surgery on another area of the face—a receding chin or pouches under the eyes—and who in the course of conversation mention the possibility of "pinning back" large and protruding ears, a condition that may have grown into a lifelong obsession.

Recently there have been some important advances in ear reconstruction that have been employed where the ears have been burned or partially destroyed, or are congenitally missing. A New Hampshire physician, Dr. Rayford Tanzer, has described the technique of reconstructing the missing or partially deformed ear by using the patient's own bone and cartilage. Dr. Tanzer takes the sixth, seventh, and eighth ribs where they come together to form the breastbone.

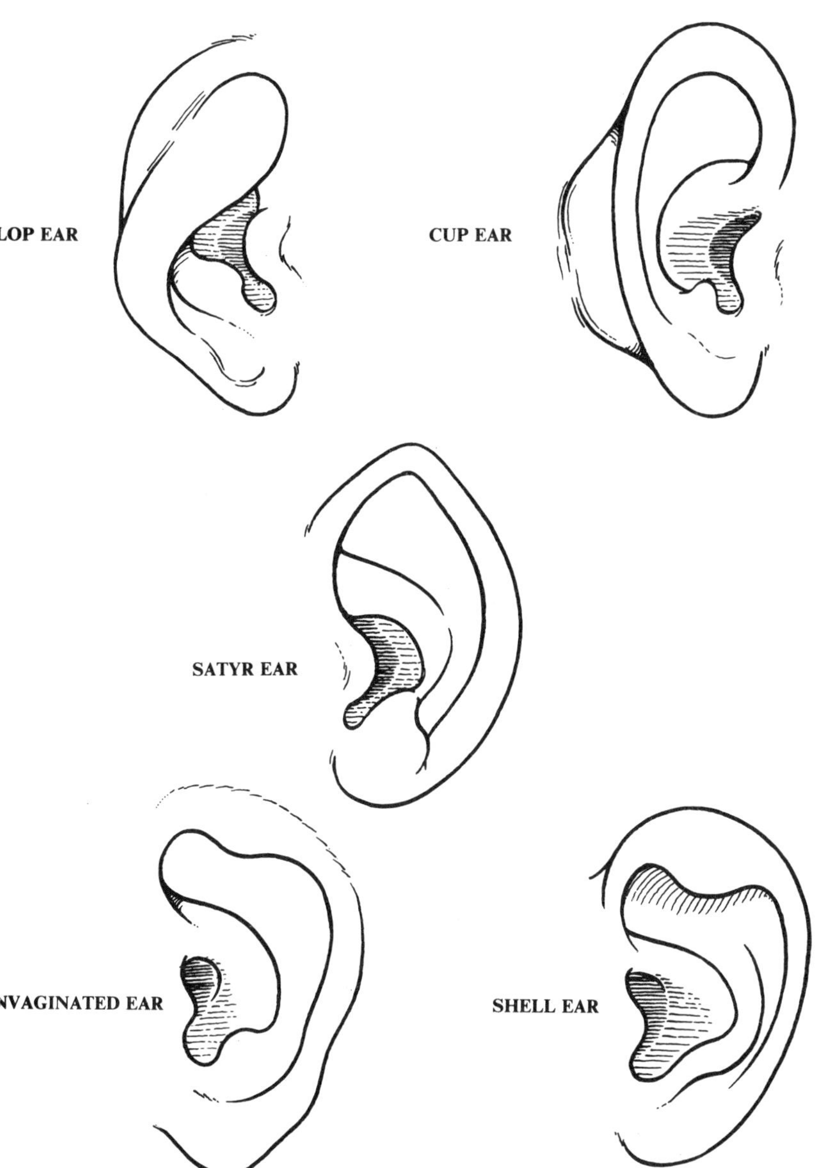

Some of the common varieties of ear deformity that can be corrected by plastic surgery

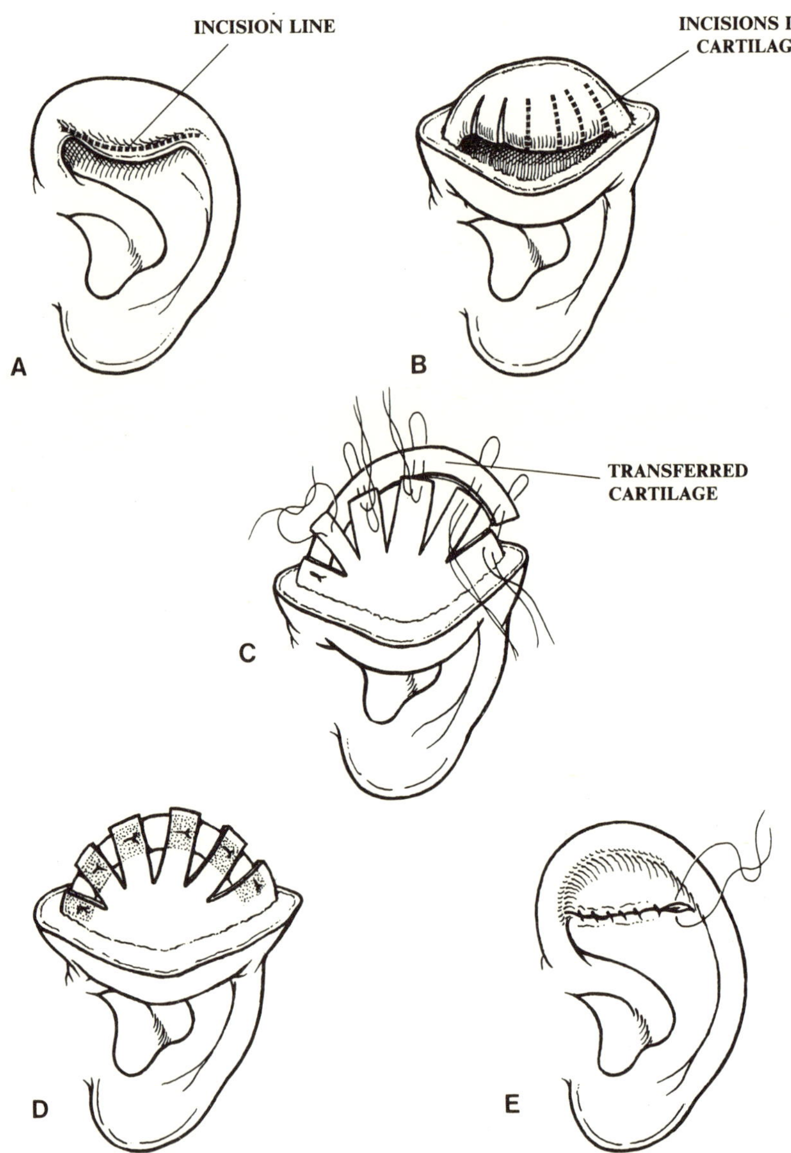

Lop Ear Correction (Otoplasty)

A. The cup ear deformity showing the line of surgical incision.
B. The folding cartilage is exposed.
C. The vertical cuts through the deformed cartilage allow it to be unfolded and sutured to a semi-lunar piece of cartilage.
D. The cartilage suturing completed.
E. Final skin suturing and the result.

The confluence of these ribs forms a long and wide source of material that can be shaved and carved with woodworking tools into proper ear-cartilage shape. This cartilagenous form is placed under the skin; subsequent operations are then necessary for the skin with underlying cartilage to be lifted forward. A final procedure projects the new ear forward so that it is not plastered against the head. A skin graft is necessary here. The advanced technique of using a patient's own body for reconstruction material is a positive one, for you do not have to deal with foreign matter, such as Silastic. Generally, I feel that whenever you can avoid placing Silastic in the body you're far better off. For example, if you're hit on the ear, the skin might be bruised and, with Silastic beneath, you might get an infection and then need a second operation to replace the implant. This is avoided by using your own available cartilage, which can handle potential infections better.

Protruding ears are the major reason men come to my office for specific ear surgery. But there are more complicated operations necessary that I and other surgeons must also perform. An entire ear may have to be constructed because a person was born without one, or has lost one to cancer or through injury. There are actually several causes of ear deformities; some have been associated with diseases, such as rubella (German measles). There are also genetic factors—if your father was endowed with protruding or pointy ears, it's likely that yours may have a similar appearance. Similarly, some ear deformities are inherited, and if both parents have them then the offspring will more than likely inherit some form of them. Most deformities can be successfully treated. However, the most common ear problems I see are those associated with some form of protrusion.

Plastic surgery can be performed on the ears of relatively young patients. So one would think that most operations would be performed on youngsters at a time when they haven't yet been taunted too much about "Dumbo" or "lop ears." Nonetheless, I treat a great many men who are in their twenties or thirties. They often tell me they had discussed their problem with their parents, who didn't think they needed an operation or else didn't want to spend the money for it. Now that these men are adults and have both a choice and their own bank accounts, they often choose to undergo the operation they've always wanted.

CASE HISTORIES

One patient in his early twenties who comes to mind is Olly R., an engineering student from Norway. He wanted to have surgery before he returned home. Olly's ears weren't misshapen, but he did feel that they were protruding too much. When I first met him his long blond hair camouflaged his ears, but Olly explained he wanted to have the option to wear his hair in a short style.

The operation lasted about forty-five minutes and involved local anesthesia, so that the patient was fully aware of what was going on. So aware, in fact, that he wanted to make sure that his ears were being pinned back closely enough to his head. Olly was concerned that he wouldn't be coming back to the United States for a while and wouldn't be able to get an adjustment soon after the surgery if he thought it was necessary. As a result, after I did one ear I showed him the results in a mirror. He looked pleased, but commented, "I wish you would bring it back a bit more." He was bothered because the lobule was still sticking out. I was able to take additional skin off from behind the ear to bring the lobule in. After this adjustment he was completely satisfied.

Dressings were placed on the young Norwegian's head and he went home an hour later. After five days I took the dressings off. The ears were a bit swollen and slightly discolored, but Olly left for Norway that same afternoon. The stitches were left, either to dissolve or be taken out by a surgeon in his native country.

I recently operated on Charles O'P, an eight-year-old boy (who of course came in with his parents). He was quite good looking but had a problem with his ears: the concha, or cuplike area of the ear, was sticking out. So in spite of a handsome face Charles had an Alfred E. Neuman appearance. The boy had brought this to his parents' attention on many occasions because he felt that people were making fun of him. After the operation, when the bandages came off, the boy saw the results and he was delighted. Best of all, his ears will remain perfect for the rest of his life.

Another case of otoplasty involves Peter G., a young actor who became my patient. Not working very regularly, he decided it was his

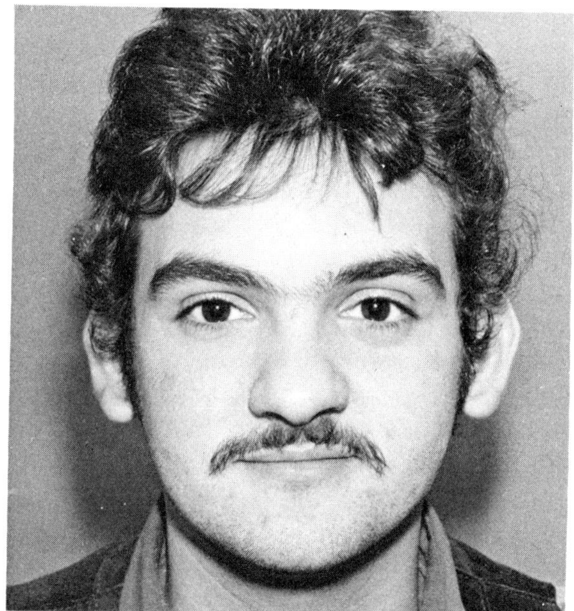

PRE-OP

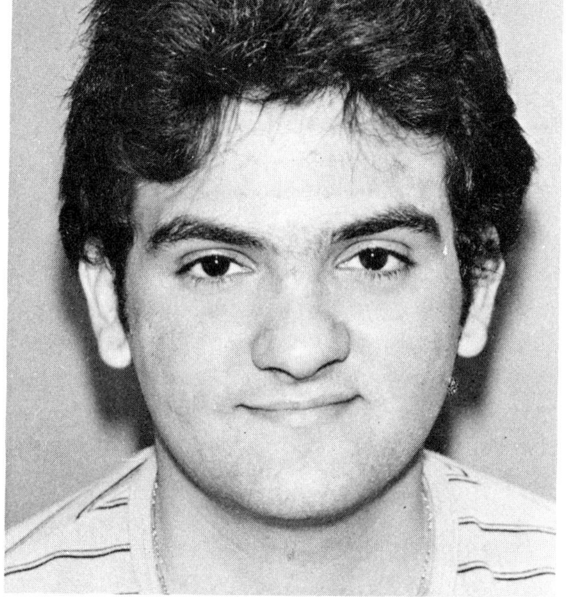

POST-OP

Ear Surgery (Otoplasty)

ears that were holding him back from his "big break." I suppose Pete didn't know about Clark Gable's success in spite of protruding ears. At any rate, I operated on him recently and the surgery has helped Peter's appearance and his view of himself. Whether it lands him leading roles or not remains to be seen.

Still another patient in my care was Aake C., a tall Swedish-American. For some reason, many Swedes seem to have big ears, and in this case Aake, who was six feet seven inches tall, had enormous ears—ears far too large even for his big face. The operation that was performed was far more complicated than most. First of all, the ears were set back because they were sticking out. Then, because of a wrong fold, they were refolded. And finally, because of the large lobules, they were cut down. Aake's ears, thanks to the operation, are now proportional to his face and body.

SELF-EVALUATION

A self-evaluation test comes down, simply, to asking yourself just how you feel about your ears. Do they bother you? Will you feel better about yourself if they're changed? Men come to my office for ear surgery not because it will help their hearing—obviously plastic surgery cannot do this—but because it can help their appearance, to others and to themselves.

BEFORE SURGERY

Otoplasty can take place in the hospital or your surgeon's office. An adult or a mature adolescent, say twelve or thirteen years old, can tolerate the procedure, and I'll do it with local anesthesia and good sedation, frequently on an outpatient basis. The operation only takes an hour and the patient generally goes home the same day. But if the patient is only seven years old, no matter how calm and "mature" he seems, he probably will have a general anesthetic, usually in the hospital.

THE PROCEDURE

Most men elect to have surgery upon their ears because the ears are not properly folded. More specifically, the helix (the rim) and the anti-helix (the subadjacent area) don't have the normal embryological folding that the majority of people have. The ears therefore are bowl shaped and look very prominent. The operation to correct this condition is not complicated. Incisions are made behind the ear, the cartilage is scored to weaken it, and then stitches are put in so that folds can be created where they should have been.

Another common complaint is that while ears are reasonably well proportioned and folded, they stick out too much at the side of the head. In other words, the ears are basically normal, but the concha, or cup, is very deep. For these men I make an incision behind the ear and cut right down to the mastoid bone, which is the bone behind the ear. I open the skin down to the cartilage, attach the cartilage to the bone, and pin the whole thing back. By "pinning" I mean taking a stitch and putting it through the upper layer of the bone, or the periosteum, which covers the bone, and then another stitch through the cartilage. Then I adjust and tighten the ear into position and put several additional stitches in to hold it back securely. That's all that has to be done. No incision is made in the concha. Operations to fold back the helix and anti-helix, as well as this particular technique that pins back the ears, usually take no more than an hour. So you can see that the problem with protruding ears is in their supporting structure—the cartilage. Many a child has had his ears taped back by a well-meaning mother, but nothing less than the reshaping of the cartilage can be permanently effective.

There are also less common procedures. For example, there's the "lop" ear, so called because a downward fold of the top of the ear makes it lop over. To correct it I remove a wedge of cartilage at the angle of the bend and then stitch the sides of the wedge to bring the upper halves of the ear into a vertical position. In refashioning the pointy, or satyr ear, the pointed section can be trimmed into a rounded shape.

Indeed, surgical corrections are available for virtually every type of ear deformity. Protruding or improperly contoured ears are taken care of easily and regularly. More complex procedures, such as total reconstruction, are also possible. In about one out of every 20,000 births a baby is born without one or both outer ears; this condition is known as microtia, a condition correctible by modern plastic surgery.

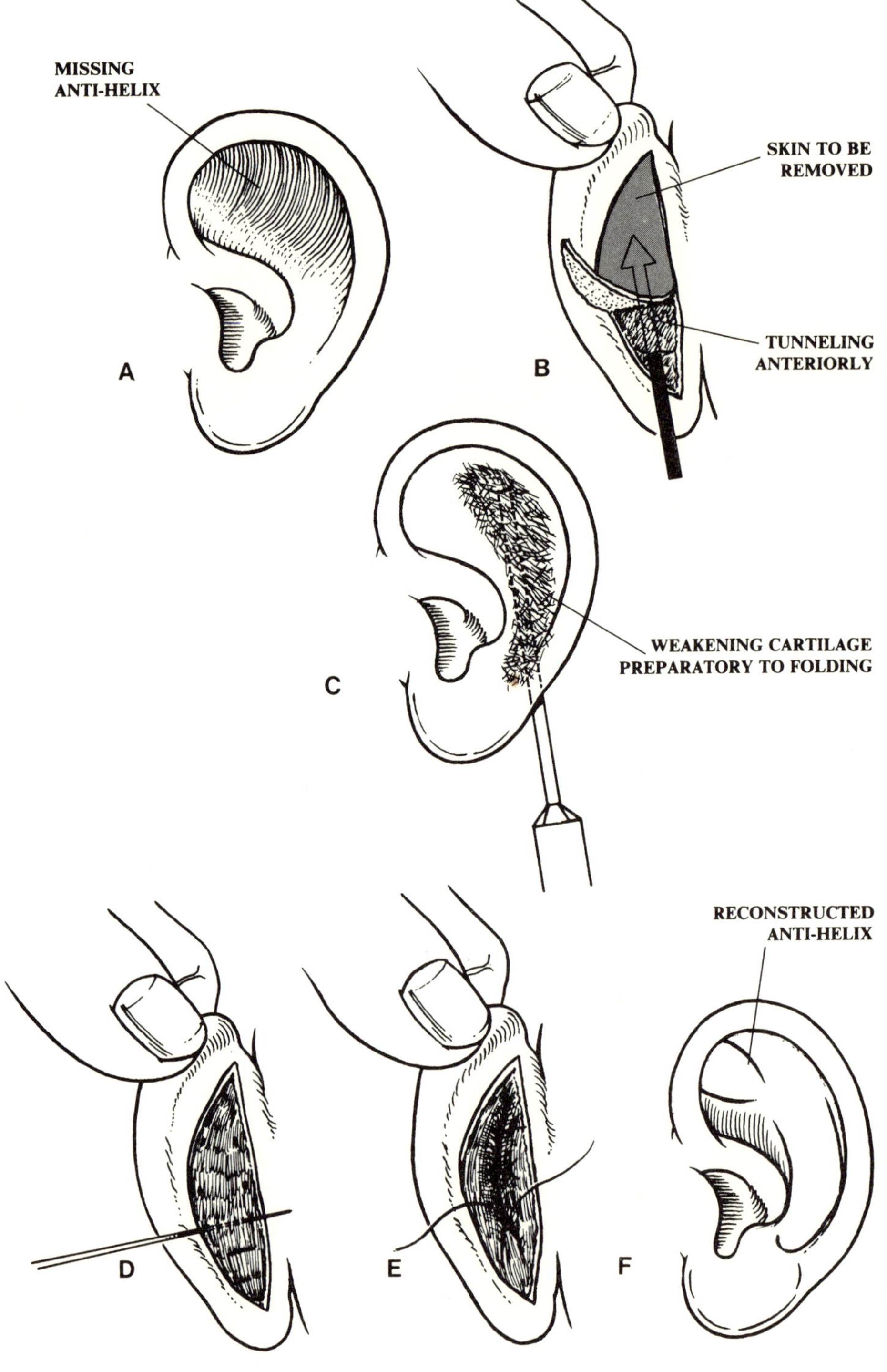

MISSING ANTI-HELIX
A
SKIN TO BE REMOVED
TUNNELING ANTERIORLY
B
WEAKENING CARTILAGE PREPARATORY TO FOLDING
C
RECONSTRUCTED ANTI-HELIX
D
E
F

Ears can be severed in accidents or destroyed because of disease. In some cases the ear can be reconstructed and in others a prosthetic ear would be advisable, because of the number of procedures necessary to complete the reconstruction. One of my patients was in a car accident and had part of his ear ripped off. I was able to reconstruct the ear by using a piece of cartilage from the opposite one, a small piece of rib, and some of the available skin in the local area. The part that was missing—the upper third of the ear—was reconstructed and looks very close to normal.

There also have been many cases of reimplantation of an avulsed, or torn, part of the ear; a reimplantation of a totally avulsed ear has also been achieved. If a major blood vessel can be found and the operation is done soon enough, and if the tissue is not severely crushed, a procedure called microvascular anastomosis may be employed to reattach the severed ear. It is often worth trying to reattach the entire ear if circumstances are conducive to the situation.

If, say, half an ear is cut off, the cartilage can be saved by preserving it. This is done by removing the skin and actually burying the cartilage under the skin of the patient's abdomen. A month or so later, it can be implanted and used again to reconstruct the ear. Using the cartilage a person is born with makes for an easier and more satisfactory operation; more so than having to sculpt a portion of an ear from a rib or other source of cartilage.

Major reconstruction will be unnecessary for all but a few. The only reason I mention it is to indicate that it is done, and to contrast

Opposite page: Treatment of the most common ear deformity

A. The normal folding of the outer portions of the ear is missing. This is the so-called "lop ear" deformity.

B. The incision is made behind the ear and a strip of excess skin is removed.

C. The stiffened non-convoluted cartilage is weakened from behind to allow for easy folding.

D. The area to be folded is outlined and held temporarily with a straight pin.

E. The permanent sutures are placed and tied to form the new shape.

F. The reconstructed ear.

such techniques with relatively simple cosmetic procedures that are performed almost every day on the ear.

AFTER SURGERY

After the operation your surgeon will apply a moistened cotton dressing that is contoured and shaped to correspond to the new ear structure; a secondary dressing is placed around the head and also around both ears.

About a week after surgery the outer dressing is changed and the contour dressing is removed. Sutures are removed at that time also, unless they are the self-dissolving type.

I usually recommend that a patient wear a ski-band type of protection at night for several weeks after surgery. It keeps the ear in position and protects it from being distorted while the patient is sleeping. It also provides a feeling of security; with the area protected, the patient is more relaxed.

The ears are usually swollen for a couple of weeks after surgery and you may experience a slight discoloration for a week or two. You can wash your hair soon after surgery. Don't, however, expose your ears to violent temperature extremes and avoid a sunburn for at least a month after the operation. If you live in an area of extreme cold, I suggest that you take special precautions by wearing a ski-type knit band when you go outdoors. It will make you feel more comfortable.

Opposite page: Total Reconstruction of the Ear

- *A. An example of microtia, or missing external ear. A small remnant of the lobe is usually all that is present.*
- *B. The cartilage framework for the reconstructed ear is carved from the flexible part of the rib cage, in the area where the breast bone and ribs meet.*
- *C. The carved framework is placed beneath the skin on the side of the head.*
- *D. Stitches are placed through the skin to cause it to adhere to the shaped cartilage framework.*
- *E. Several months after Step D, the newly formed ear is given projection from the side of the head by placing a skin graft behind it to elevate it from the scalp.*

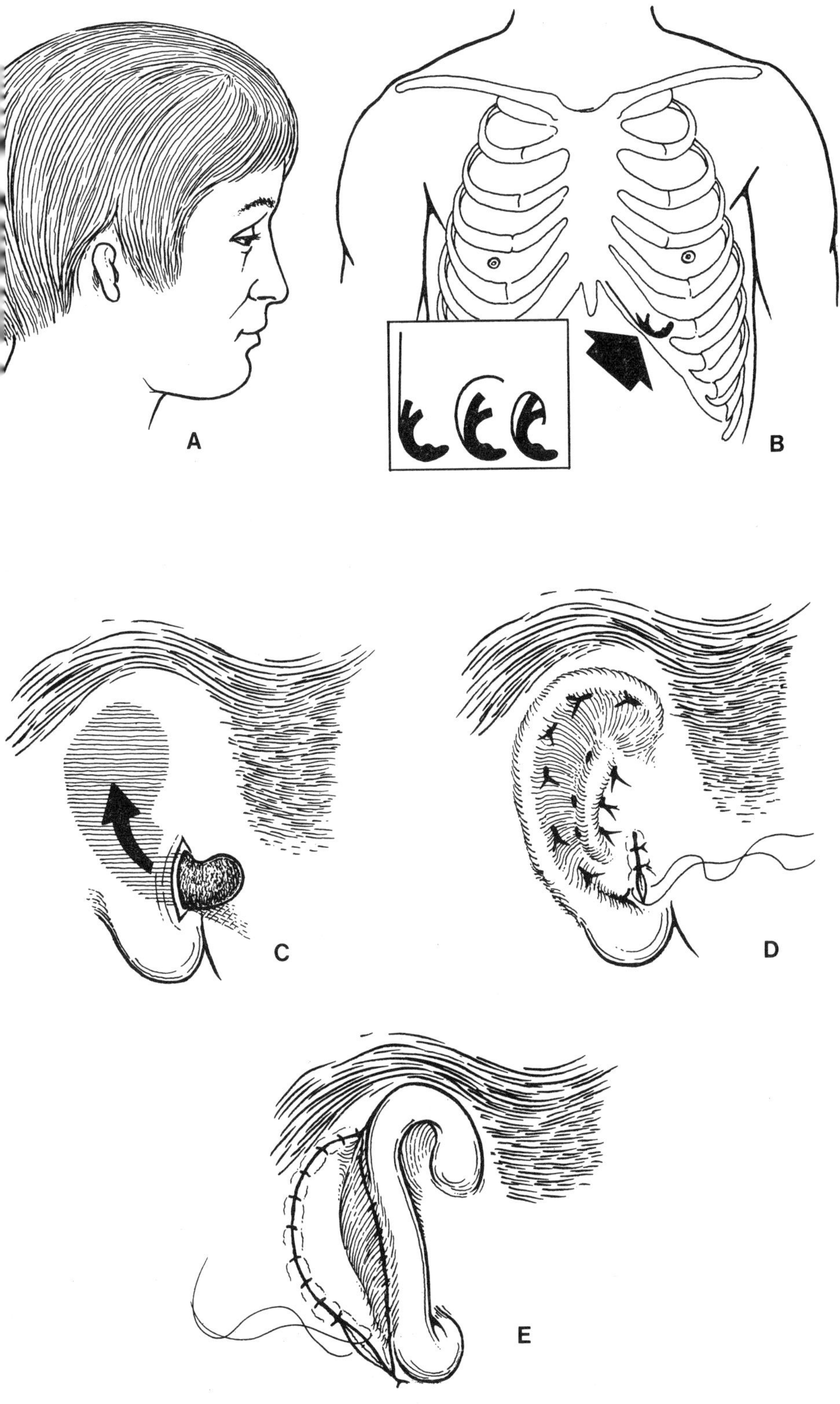
A
B
C
D
E

WHAT CAN GO WRONG

Complications from otoplasty are unusual, but they do occur. If for some reason an infection develops, it is easily treated with antibiotics. It is possible that when the incision is closed up blood may accumulate beneath the skin, because there is a potential dead space where the cartilage is separated from the skin. The presence of blood may be indicated by unusual pain while the postoperative dressing is on. If such is the case, the doctor will remove the dressing, make a small incision, and remove the accumulated blood by draining it. The ear can then be recontoured with a compression dressing. As an interesting side light, if the ear is subject to repeated injury, such as with a boxer, fluid and blood accumulate and a tremendous amount of scar tissue can occur. The ear becomes distorted and the so-called "cauliflower" ear results.

Keloids, or scars that keep on growing in a sort of overhealing process, can also be a postoperative problem. Some people are susceptible to keloids after incisions are made, and end up with enormous keloid growth at the operative site. So if I know that a man is subject to keloids I will not operate—not even behind the ears. The various treatments for keloids—radiation, compression therapy, injections of steroids—don't always work.

WHAT YOU CAN EXPECT

The end result of cosmetic surgery of the ear is always in proportion to the original problem. A relatively simple situation like a protruding ear should give good results when the ear is otherwise well formed. Ears that are pointy or don't have the proper folds, ears with minor-part deficiencies such as missing lobules, will also have the best results if the congenital abnormality is not severe.

Most cosmetic ear surgery strives for as natural looking an ear as possible—an ear neither too far away nor too close to the head. What is not desirable are sharp edges of cartilage or unnatural irregularities of the ear framework. If minor irregularities of contour do develop, they can be treated by a minor secondary operation. (Keep in mind, however, that no two ears are the same; so don't expect them to be exact mirror images after surgery.)

Also, as I have already said, don't assume that alterations in your appearance will radically alter your life. Cosmetic surgery is not meant to open up the windows of the world, or to conquer new ones. What plastic surgery on the ears can and does do is correct a problem that may have disturbed your emotional state and peace of mind, so that a new self-confidence may emerge—one that will allow you to get more out of life.

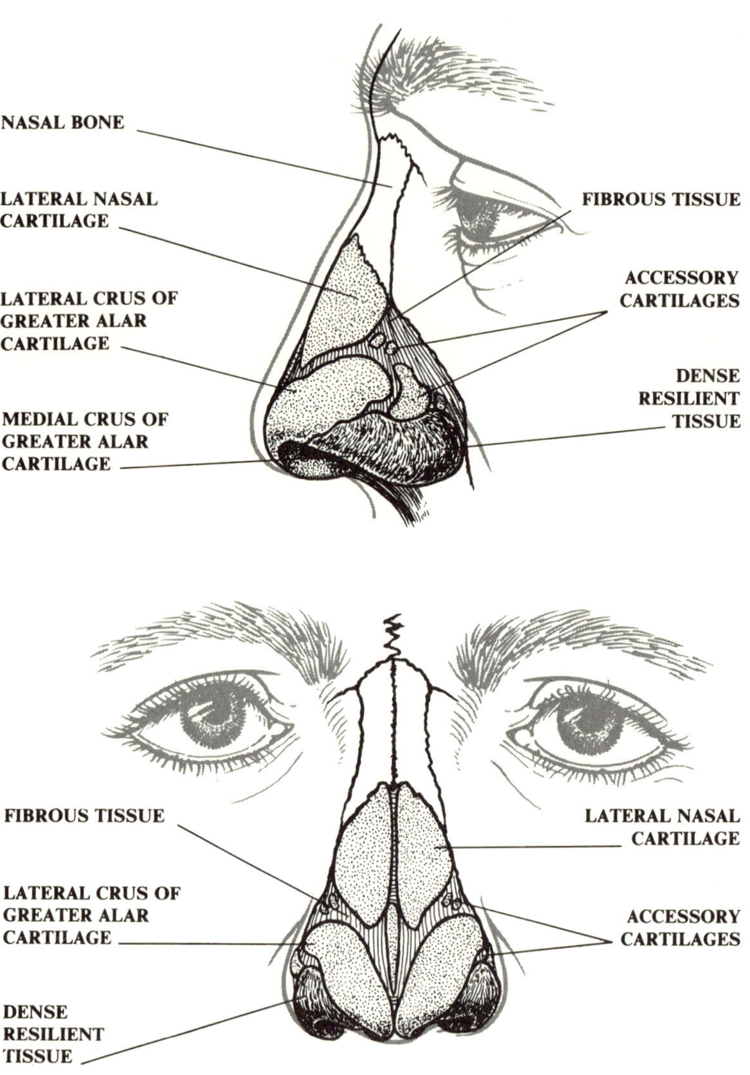

The Anatomy of the Nose

A. The nose in profile showing the cartilaginous and bony structures which help to form and support it.

B. A front view of the supporting bone and cartilage framework of the nose.

EIGHT

Rhinoplasty: The Nose

BECAUSE America is a nation of immigrants, a melting pot where many ethnic and genetic factors influence the shape of the nose and the face on which it sits, there really is no such characteristic feature as an "American nose." What may be considered a perfect nose for one face would be wrong for another. The only valid standard for the shape of a nose and its esthetic appeal is whether the nose proportionally fits the face. Scale and balance have a great deal to do with the overall visual effect. When a nose is inappropriate, when it is too large for the face and dominates the features, the effect will not be harmonious. From Cyrano to Pinocchio to Quasimodo, a nose that distorts the rest of the face can not only dominate an individual's expression, but may also affect his self-esteem.

Since the shape of the nose is influenced by genetics, one's ethnic background is identified often more by the nose than by any other single feature. We refer to a Mediterranean, an African, an Oriental, and a Roman nose. There was a time when a second-generation American with an ethnic nose might have considered it a handicap, but today, when we stress ethnic pride and purity, a nose that may identify one's heritage is not necessarily undesirable. In fact, some of the male models who dominate the fashion ads have more than generous noses, far wider and less perfect than the old idea of what was handsome. An actor with a battered fighter's nose is considered "sexy" by his female fans; the nose is a part of his he-man image. The not-quite-perfect nose is considered attractive today.

The look that seems most desirable is a natural one. Today's man seeks a nose that is in proportion to the rest of his face, one that fits his concept of how he would like to look and how he wants the world to see him.

THE ANATOMY OF A NOSE

Needless to say, there is more to a nose than only its esthetic character; it must also be functional. It is made up of a few small bones, some cartilage, skin on the outside, and mucous membrane on the inside. A septum of cartilage divides the nose into right and left portions. The nose forms the beginning of the respiratory tract. Air filtered through hairs at the opening of the nostrils is warmed and moistened before it reaches the throat and larynx and lungs. The sense of smell is transmitted to the brain by nerve endings located in the upper portion of the mucous membrane. The nose also affects voice quality, through resonance.

Surgery on the nose can be performed for cosmetic as well as for functional reasons—sometimes at the same time. A single operation can make a patient look better and also allow him to breathe easier, as, for instance, when a deviated septum needs correction. Not every deviated septum, however, is the cause of obstructive breathing, which may also be caused by allergies to pollen, dust, and a variety of other elements. The patient who has allergies and expects his breathing to be improved by an operation that corrects his septum may be in for a disappointment.

CASE HISTORIES

While there is no typical person who comes to me for rhinoplasty, those who do reflect the openness and candor of today's cosmetic surgery. The men are of all ages and occupations and come to see me for a wide range of reasons. Some are models or actors, men who are always keenly aware of their appearance. Then there are the professionals and businessmen who are displeased with this one aspect of their appearance and have decided to do something about it.

One patient of mine had a particularly unusual background for someone consulting a New York doctor. Alexander was a native of Greece who was studying at an Italian medical school. He came to my office because he had heard from a doctor cousin of his in the Midwest about the outpatient surgery I perform.

This Greek medical student was a striking looking young man—all six feet eight inches of him. In addition to studying medicine,

Alex was also doing part-time work as an actor. Being able to speak several languages had helped him land some minor roles in international films. He was very handsome, but he also had a very large nose, which had what is best described as a high takeoff from the forehead; it seemed to come directly out, in the style of the classic nose seen on ancient coins and statues. This wasn't Alex's problem, though, at least not in how he saw himself. The problem was an enormous bump on the nose. Alex was anxious that an operation not change the ethnicity of his nose. I assured him that I was also interested in a natural looking nose, which meant taking off the bump while not changing the high takeoff from his forehead. (Had he requested it, however, it would have been possible for me to have deepened the angle just a bit more at the point where the nose protrudes from the forehead.)

The rhinoplasty was performed along with a secondary procedure—a slight lengthening of the upper lip, which had been elevated because of the bump. Soon after the surgery, Alexander returned to school in Italy. He came back to see me during the Christmas recess, six months after the operation had been performed. All the swelling was down and the nose was in proportion to his face. We were both quite pleased with the results.

Another patient of mine was Ray F., an twenty-two-year-old college student, who was quite intelligent but had some personal adjustment problems. Apparently, he was somewhat of a recluse. Part of his problem had to do with self-consciousness about his nose. Ray came to see me on referral from his family physician.

I didn't have to look too closely to observe that the young man had a twisted and ungainly nose that just didn't fit his face. It was a congenital deformity; all the parts of the nose were there but the cartilage was misshapen, giving the appearance of a twisted long nose. There was also a considerable protuberance, or bump.

During the rhinoplasty the bump was removed. Ray's nose itself was straightened out by making the nasal bones symmetrical on both sides. Extensive cartilage at the tip of the nose itself was also distorting it, and so a large portion of the cartilage was taken out. Of course, some cartilage had to be left for supportive purposes; otherwise the nose would collapse like a tent with the poles taken out.

The cast came off in a week and the improvement in Ray's ap-

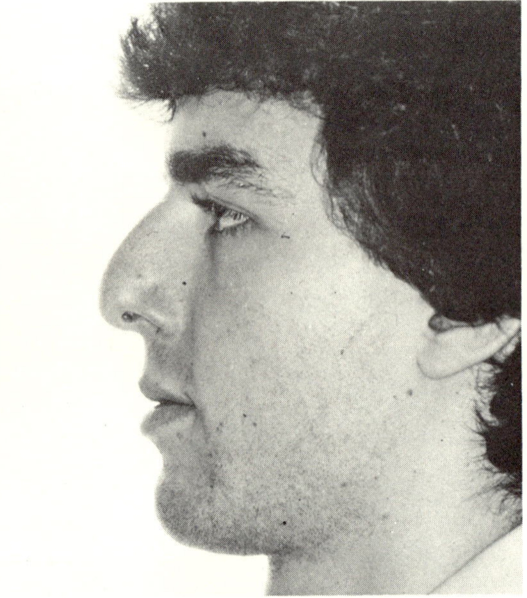

BEFORE

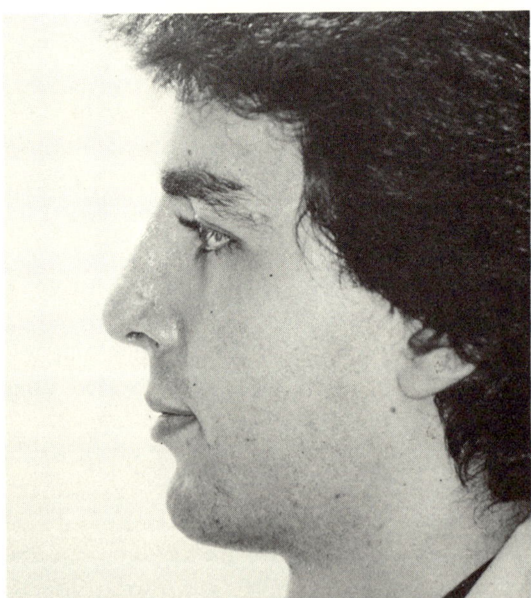

AFTER

Nose Surgery (Rhinoplasty)—Before and After

pearance was strikingly evident. When he came back for a second postoperative visit he looked even better. That's because he had a new haircut and was obviously showing more care and interest in his clothes. In fact, he seemed far more affable and outgoing. The physical and mental improvement in this case was so obvious that I couldn't help but wonder why he waited so long to have the operation performed.

Not every patient falls into the schoolboy category. A recently divorced forty-two-year-old man comes to mind. When Jason F. first consulted me, I could see that he was fairly content, a successful businessman, well dressed, and good looking by most standards. Jason felt, however, that his nose was too prominent because of a slight twist. In this case, he didn't want a newly shaped nose to help him achieve success; he had already reached most of his goals. He simply thought that his nose was disproportionate to the rest of his good features and wanted it corrected. I performed the minor corrections, and today Jason feels that he looks better for having decided to undergo the surgery.

Another patient of mine, in his mid-forties, was unhappy with a nose that was both long and twisted. Jack L. had no illusions of an operation changing his life or lifestyle. He was unmarried, had a job he liked as a cabinetmaker, and supported his aged mother and father. In this case, Jack was an average individual who wanted to improve his appearance. The operation was performed and he was pleased. Jack made no apparent attempt to change his way of life because of his new appearance—he didn't, for example, become a Don Juan, on the prowl for women in the singles bars. He continued to take care of his parents and to go to work every day as he had prior to his rhinoplasty. However, he felt better with what he considered a "perfect" nose. And, now, Jack is scheduled for a face-lift. Obviously improving his looks has made him a happier man.

Not every patient walks out of my office enraptured. One teenager who came to see me had already had rhinoplasty performed by another surgeon. He wanted me to redo it. He thought the entire world was staring at his "prizefighter's" nose. I didn't see anything wrong with his nose, except for perhaps a slight thickness at the tip. An operation would have resulted in very little improvement at best, and

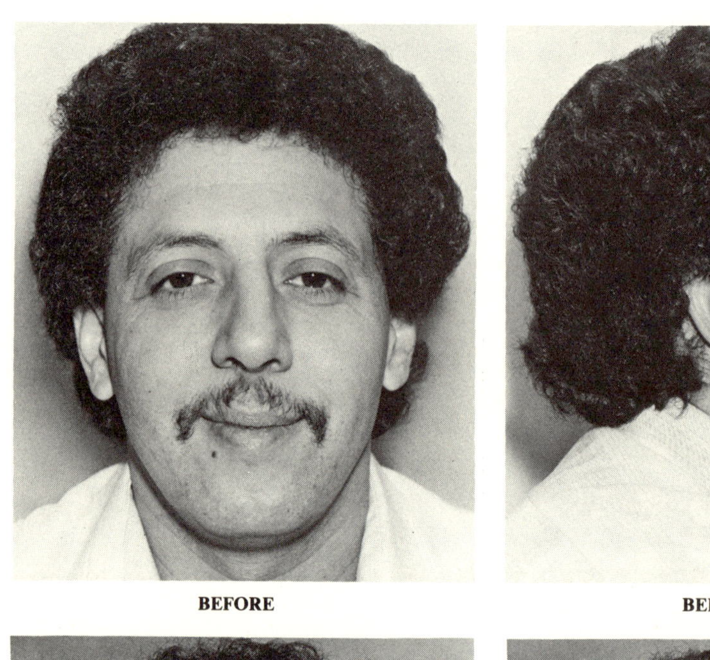

BEFORE BEFORE

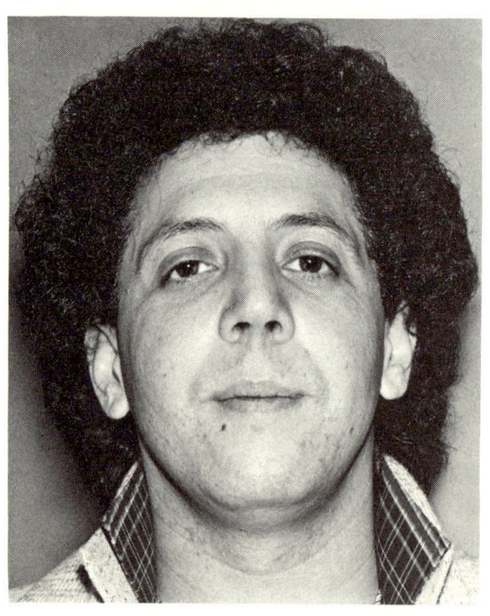

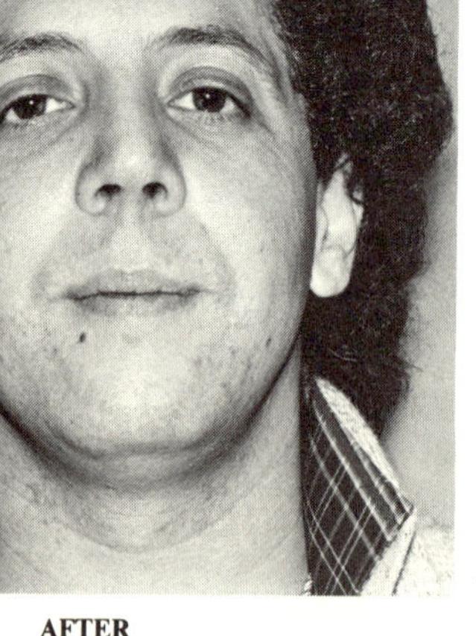

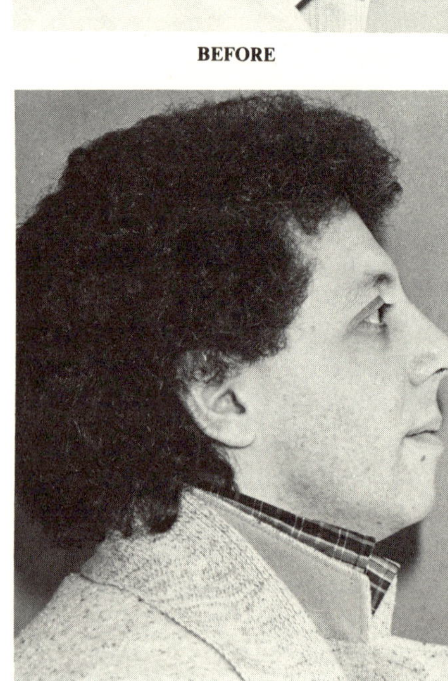

AFTER AFTER

Nose Surgery—Before and After

the patient, I felt, would even then be dissatisfied. So I would not perform the surgery.

This teenager happened to be under the care of a psychiatrist. I would, and do, perform surgery on patients under psychiatric care when there is something wrong with the nose and the psychiatrist recommends surgery. Very often cosmetic surgery can help remove psychological blocks. But when a patient with an otherwise normal nose insists the world is staring at it and at him, an operation is obviously not going to improve his emotional health.

SELF-EVALUATION

Your decision to seek corrective nasal surgery is usually made long before your first consultation with a plastic surgeon. You have already become aware—perhaps painfully—that there is some aspect of your nose that you're unhappy with. You see it every day in the mirror when you're shaving. Someone may have made unkind comments about your nose, and you feel that it is not your most flattering feature. The question "Do I need the surgery?" usually has an obvious answer.

The Age Factor

The earliest time you should consider rhinoplasty is in your late teens—at seventeen or eighteen years of age. While a female can have the surgery performed a year or two earlier, a male may still have a growth spurt at age seventeen. If the operation is performed before full growth is attained, a slight overgrowth of the nasal bones may occur following such a growth spurt, partially negating the good result of the operation. However, if a youngster really has a psychological problem because of his nose, an operation may be performed earlier. In this case, if a minor revision is required, it can be taken care of later on.

It might seem a bit strange for a man over fifty to seek rhinoplasty, yet there are many men in an older age category who say, "This hook has always bothered me and even though I'm getting older I want to have it taken care of." This, in my opinion, is a valid reason to have rhinoplasty performed. Naturally, a man of any age who has an automobile accident or trauma is also a candidate for the surgery. In addition, anyone who has a blockage of the nose as the result of a deviated septum may elect surgery to improve his breathing.

BEFORE SURGERY

While you may think you already know a great deal about rhinoplasty through reading or learning of the experiences of friends, your first consultation with a plastic surgeon is still quite important. You will want to ask questions of him, to gain confidence that he is expert enough to do the kind of work you want. He will want to learn about you as well, particularly whether your wishes and expectations are realistic and within the realm of the possible.

At the consultation the doctor is apt to ask what it is that bothers you. If you answer, "I just don't like the way I look," he may become a bit wary. He will be less apprehensive if you state in more definite terms just what it is you are dissatisfied with; otherwise, he will believe that you want more than your nose reshaped, that perhaps you want to change your whole life.

I take photographs of a patient's nose from several angles—generally of both profiles, one with the patient smiling, and one aimed upwards at the tip of the nose. I want the patient to see his nose as it really is and not how he may think it looks. The patient then usually points out how he would like his nose changed, and I can give him some idea of the outcome that is possible with surgery. If there are certain desired changes that can't be made, these too are discussed fully.

The surgeon, no matter how skilled, is limited in the degree of the changes that he can accomplish. One limiting factor is the thickness and quality of the skin—if a man's nasal skin is thick, the most facile chiseling and sculpturing will not show up as well as if it were thin. Likewise, if a nose is very large it can't be made too small—if you remove too much bone on a big nose there is the problem of what to do with all the excess skin, for it can shrink just so much, resulting in a distorted appearance.

In other words, don't buy a copy of the latest men's fashion magazine, look over the models, and say, "This is the nose I want." The surgeon is limited to a certain degree not only by the quality of your skin and its thickness, but by the size of the bone beneath. What you can ask for—and receive—is a modification of your nose, not a new one. In most cases, this will satisfy your needs.

The purpose of the operation is not to create a nose that looks artificial, as if it had been sculpted. You want a nose that looks natural and in proportion to the rest of your face.

I try to make clear to a patient that his nose has to be viewed as part of the entire face. In other words, what seems like a very prominent nose may just be a normal-sized one that is overly emphasized by an underdeveloped chin; perhaps it is the chin that needs the work in the first place, or done at the same time as the nose. Nasal reduction and chin augmentation are frequently performed simultaneously.

THE PROCEDURE

Most rhinoplasty takes about an hour to perform. The operation may be performed, as already mentioned, in hospital or on an outpatient basis in a doctor's facility. If you are going to have it done in the hospital, you'll be admitted the day prior to surgery, or early on the day of surgery. No matter where the surgery takes place, you'll be given some mild sedation about an hour and a half before the operation, so that you'll be relaxed and somewhat sleepy when taken to the operating room.

There, an intravenous will be started for the administration of a supplemental sedative, usually Valium, and a protective antibiotic ophthalmic ointment will be placed in your eyes. Then you'll receive a routine facial cleansing—a mild iodine solution (it doesn't burn) or pHisoHex soap to prepare the operative area.

The inside of your nose will be packed with a solution—usually a combination of cocaine and adrenalin—that numbs the nasal lining and also minimizes the oozing of blood during the operation.

After your face is prepped and draped, the surgeon injects a numbing solution of novocaine with epinephrine, which substantially reduces interoperative bleeding. You'll feel several pinpricks, and then, in almost no time at all, the entire nasal area will be anesthetized. Not only does the area become numb, but there is a shrinkage of surrounding blood vessels.

The general rhinoplasty procedure may be described as follows.

After about five or ten minutes, when the anesthetic becomes fully effective, an incision is made inside the nostril. The surgeon separates the skin from the bone underneath. This tent of skin is pulled away, with special instruments, allowing him to get to the bone and gently chisel it down. He artfully shapes and molds it, removing any disfiguring bump. The bigger the distortion that's removed, the wider the nose becomes. Therefore it is necessary to break the bones so that they can be moved in a direction that narrows the nose. This breaking is accomplished by sawing or chiseling the bone through the small incision that has previously been made within the nose.

Another procedure involves the tip—the end of the nose formed by two C-shaped cartilages that you can see and feel. The width is trimmed to about one or two millimeters from a previous three or four. In this manner the nasal tip is softened, allowing it to be more easily sculptured. In addition to being thinned out, the cartilages are brought in a bit; this is accomplished by scoring the cartilage so that the resiliency of the rim is decreased and the projection of the tip is allowed to descend.

A condition often associated with a nasal protrusion is one in which the upper lip is pulled up, sometimes exposing the upper teeth. This is caused by the skin being forced to go over the protrusion, which creates a tendency to raise the lip. Once it is cut off, there is a bit of excess skin that allows the upper lip to relax a bit. The surgeon can also cut the muscle that elevates the upper lip; a piece of cartilage can be placed there to prevent the muscle from reattaching the upper lip to the nose.

After the nose is reshaped, a splint is applied to the outside of the nose so that the new form can be maintained. This nasal splint is made of gauze impregnated with plaster that hardens when submerged in water. The splint permits the nasal bones to be molded and held into position so that the skin readheres to the underlying structure; it also keeps some of the swelling down. Although it is not weighty, the splint, which remains on for about a week, crisscrosses over the nose and may also cross over to your forehead. Obviously, it is visible.

During the procedure you will be breathing through your mouth and will continue to do so for some time after the operation because of the packing and swelling. This, however, is not any more uncomfortable than if you had mild nasal congestion.

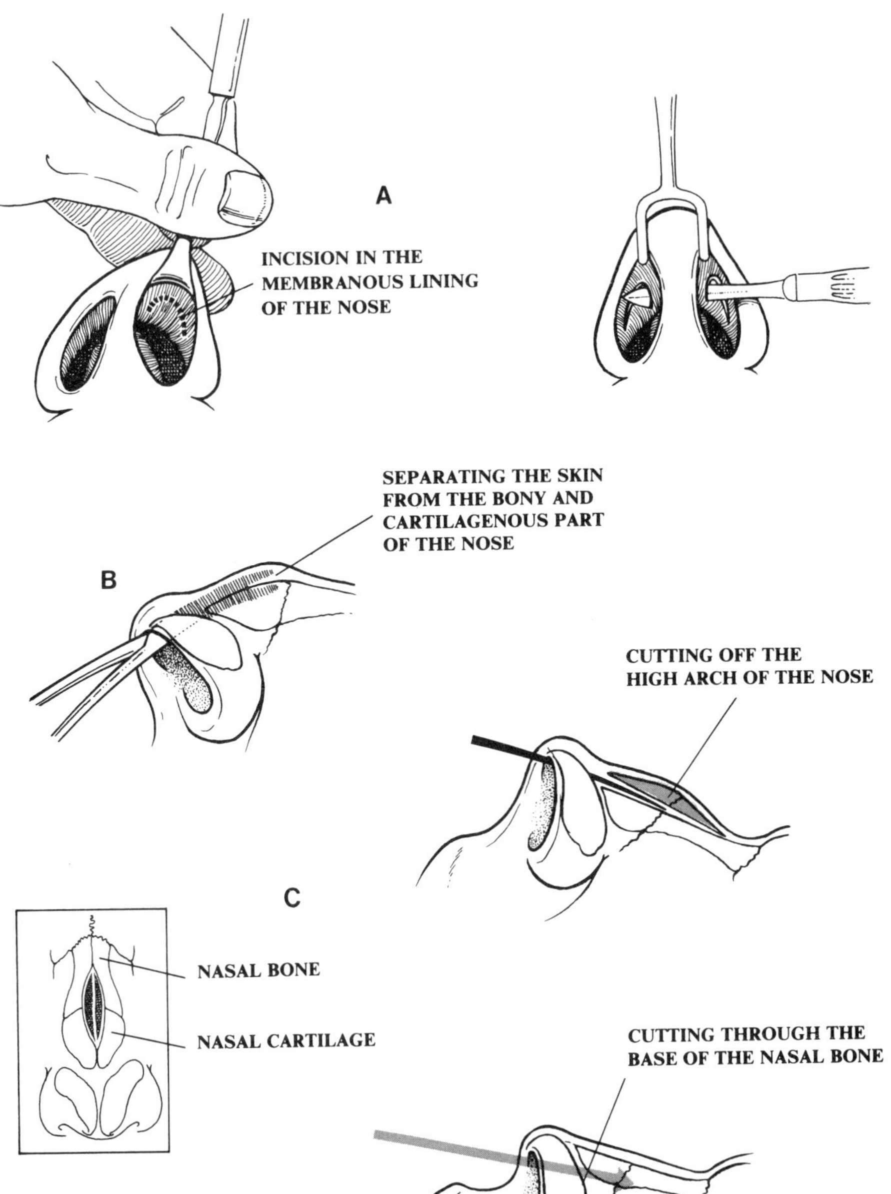

***Nose Surgery* (*Rhinoplasty*)**

A. The incision and re-shaping are done within the nose so that no external scars are made.

B. The skin is separated from the underlying nasal bones.

C. The bony hump is removed.

D. The resultant lowering of the nasal profile.

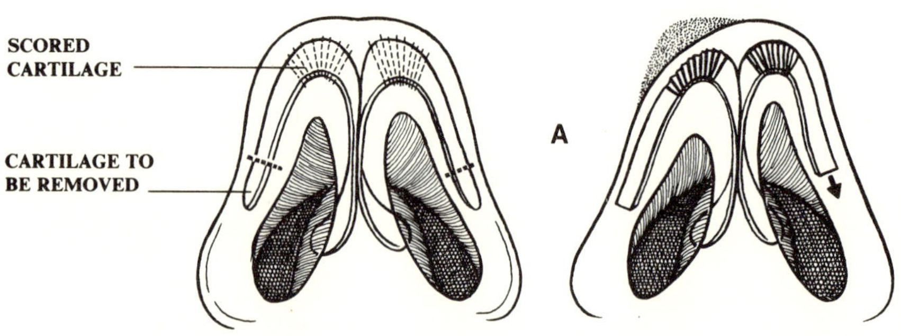

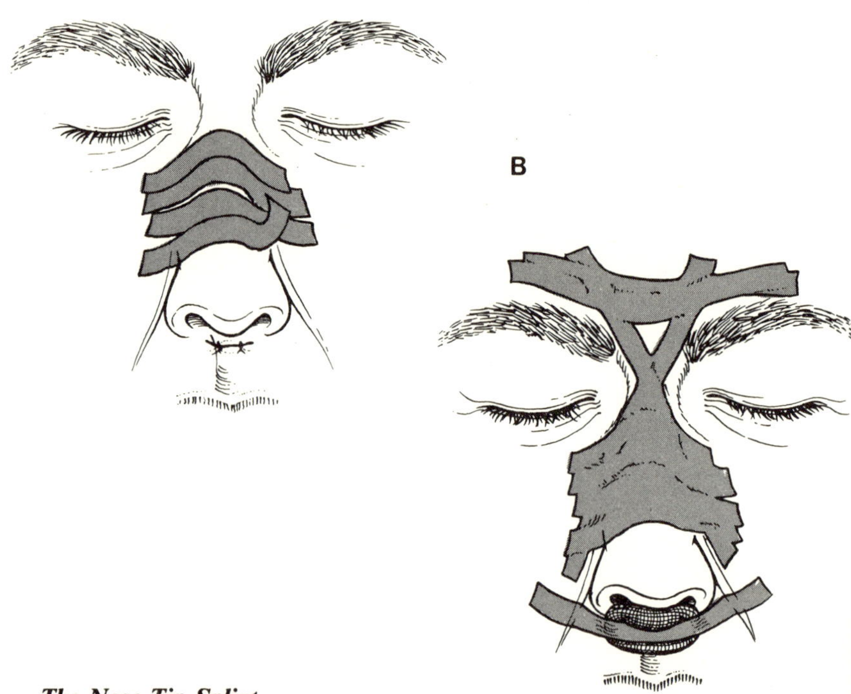

The Nose Tip Splint

A. A view of the supporting cartilages of the nasal tip. Notice the square or boxy tip caused by the cartilage. Weakening the supporting cartilage allows the nasal tip to become narrower.

B. The application of the nasal splint.

Other Procedures

Rhinoplasty performed today does not produce external scars because the corrections are accomplished internally. An exception would be the operation to modify flaring nostrils. The external incision, even in this procedure, will not leave obvious scars, for it is placed in the area where the nostrils meet the upper lip.

One other procedure that is done externally relates to the cobblestone, or W.C. Fields, type of nose. This condition has nothing to do, as commonly thought, with excessive drinking. It is caused by the overproduction of sebaceous glands—those glands that lubricate the skin. The treatment here involves taking a knife or an electrocautery and actually shaving the skin down. The surgeon can reshape the nose, being careful not to go down to the cartilage or bone, and leaving enough nasal tissue to allow for spontaneous healing without requiring skin grafting. When the surface of the nose heals, there will be some scarring and a whitish sheen that makes the skin appear a different color from the surrounding area; nevertheless, there will be considerable improvement over the previous appearance of the nose.

Not all rhinoplasty involves cutting away bone and reducing size. Some procedures involve building up the nose. This may be desirable because trauma has caused the nasal bones to be pushed down, destroying part of the septum. When the upper part of the nose is depressed, you have a condition that is called "saddle nose," which means a depression rather than a bump. Some height can be restored by cutting the bones and moving them closer together. Usually this isn't enough; something has to be placed there to fill the depression—bone, cartilage, or a Silastic strut (a contoured piece of plastic). I find an effective technique is to take available cartilage from behind the ear; this can give height to the nose. It is also possible to use a piece of rib, or even a piece of hipbone or legbone.

When it comes to building up the nose I do not like to use Silastic implants. (My objection to this has already been mentioned in connection with otoplasty.) I believe that when there is a foreign body or Silastic implant under the skin, and if the nose is touched roughly or knocked, there is the chance of extrusion and infection. No matter how skillfully you put in a plastic implant, it is possible that a little piece may protrude through the skin; it could then start to erode and break down the overlying skin.

AFTER SURGERY

After surgery you can expect some swelling and black-and-blue discoloration around your eyes, as well as a certain amount of swelling in the upper facial area. In some cases, your eyes may also appear bloodshot. There will be minor discomfort, but mild painkillers can take care of that.

Because there has been an incision and nasal bones have been broken, a certain amount of blood will ooze out of the nostrils. Packing the nose is becoming less common, because when the packing is removed bleeding usually is stimulated all over again. A drip pad may instead be placed under the nose so that postoperative oozing can be absorbed.

Some men tell me, "I panic if I can't breathe through my nose." To calm them I explain that a ventilating tube can be put in the nose. The tube, however, usually plugs up after a few days and then is easily removed, by which time a good deal of the swelling has resolved itself, allowing easier breathing.

There's no prediction as to how long your nose will remain feeling stuffed. I've had many men come back in a day or so and say they already have some air through their nostrils; most report that as the swelling starts to decrease, some air is able to get through. It's possible to clear out some obstruction with a Q-Tip, but there's the risk of stimulating bleeding when blood crusts are removed. It's better if this probing is avoided and the nose is allowed to heal by itself for about five to seven days. When the cast is off you may then clean the insides of the nostrils with a Q-Tip and some hydrogen peroxide. At that time you'll be able to breathe more normally.

When the cast is removed you will see the results of the operation. But remember that the cast has been keeping down a certain amount of the swelling and when it's off your nose may then puff up for several days. Additionally, the swelling may not reduce uniformly, so that the nose might falsely appear to be less than straight. The condition, of course, is temporary and the final results of the

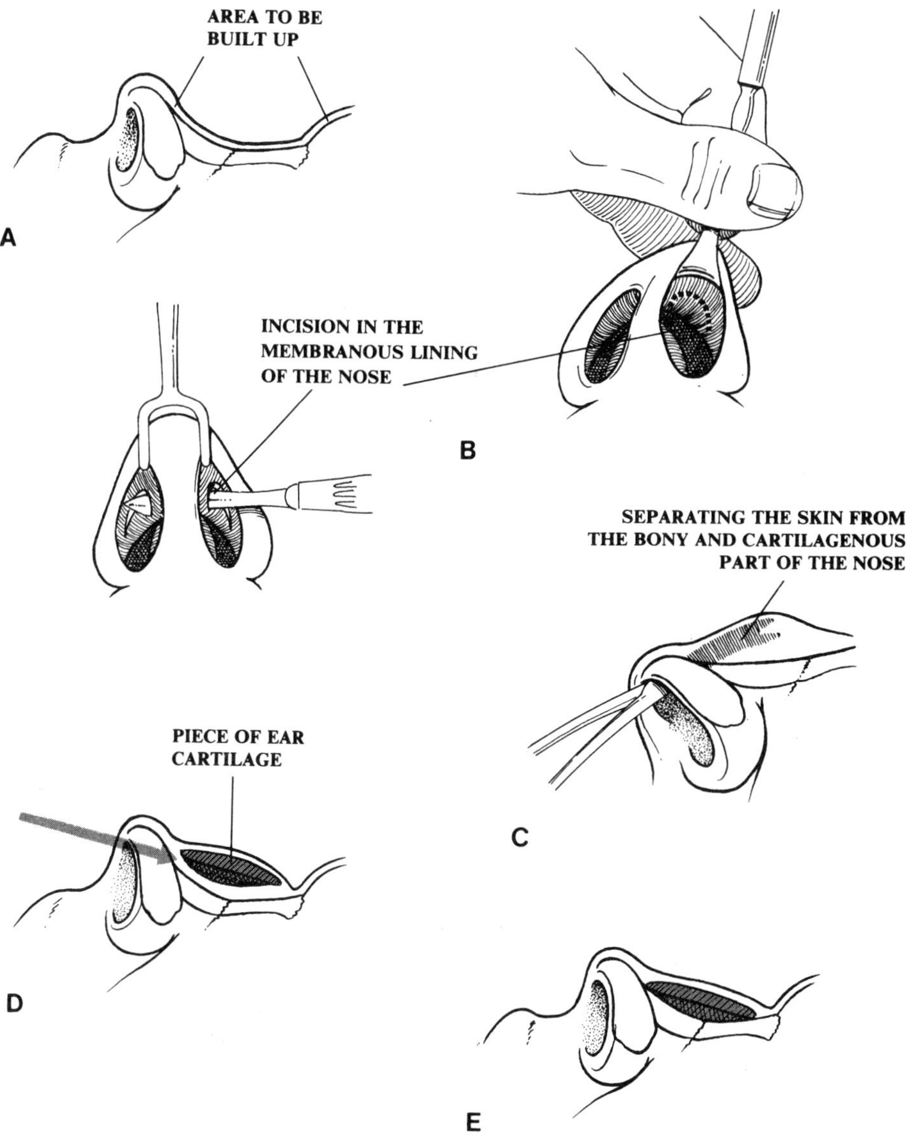

Building Up the Nose

A. The so-called "saddle-nose" deformity.

B. The incision is made entirely inside the nose.

C. The skin is separated from the underlying bone.

D. A piece of ear cartilage is used to build up the depressed area.

E. The newly formed nose.

surgeon's work will not be apparent until as long as nine months after the operation. It's important not to assume that something went wrong until everything has had a chance to heal fully, and this does take time and patience. In a small percentage of cases a minor correction may be necessary, but usually at least a year should pass after the first operation before determining whether a second one is to be undertaken.

After rhinoplasty you'll have to treat yourself tenderly. For example, you won't be able to blow your nose for the first two weeks after the operation, yet sneezing won't affect the surgery. If you wear contact lenses, you won't be able to wear them for two or three weeks following surgery. If you wear regular glasses, they should be lightweight. You may have to tape the glasses up a little, off the bridge of your nose, and place a piece of cotton there so you won't have the glasses pressing into and indenting the swollen area.

You'll probably want to wait until the cast is removed—from five to seven days after surgery—before returning to work. Your nose, of course, will still be swollen and there will be telltale black-and-blue marks about the eyes. Some men prefer to wear dark glasses until the swelling and bruised look disappear. Many, though, feel little or no embarrassment or self-consciousness.

WHAT CAN GO WRONG

One of the most difficult and unpredictable aspects of nasal surgery is the healing process. When you cut bones and break them, one side of the nose may heal differently from the other. And when the surgeon takes out the cartilage or carves and sculpts it, there may be some slight asymmetry. The nasal tip is prominent and so, if not perfect, may need minor reshaping later.

In about 8 or 10 percent of the cases some revision might be necessary. The more difficult the operation—the larger the nose, the more injured, the more twisted—the greater is the chance for a revisionary secondary procedure. When a man has straightforward cosmetic surgery and has never before had any breaks in his nose, then it becomes an easier case to handle, assuring far better results. But if the bones have been broken, twisted, and distorted, and if the bones must be rebroken, no one can safely predict how these bones are going to break. They may break along unpredictable cleavage planes and are more difficult to shape into a predictable position during the procedure.

If the nose is hit or bumped during the healing process, there can be complications. In the few cases where trauma takes place within a week or two after surgery, the nasal bones may have to be reset. Mild touching or bumping of the nose, however, rarely causes any severe or permanent damage. If you're at all concerned, have the nose examined by your surgeon. He is there to help and to reassure you.

WHAT YOU CAN EXPECT

After rhinoplasty, your face will look different and you will have a new profile. As mentioned above, it will take a substantial amount of time for the new nose to achieve its true and final shape. If you're having the operation for a special occasion, such as a college re-union or a wedding, I would suggest you plan to have it done at least two months before.

And keep in mind that there are certain characteristics of the nose that will remain unchanged; the surgeon can only work with what is there.

NINE

Mentoplasty: The Chin and Jaw

IN ANALYZING the face when contemplating possible alterations of jaw structure, three areas must be kept in mind: first, the teeth and their relationship to each other; second, the bony and soft-tissue structures, i.e., facial bones, lips, teeth, etc.; and, finally, the relationship of the upper and lower jaws to each other.

When is a jaw too far forward or too far back? This is not something that can be determined by simple visual observation but more precisely by the use of a study called cephalometrics, in which certain lines are drawn—using fixed anatomical landmarks—to determine which way the jaw needs to be moved for facial harmony.

A cephalogram—a special X ray of the skull in profile—is then taken. The cephalogram shows not only the bony structure of the head but also the soft tissues overlying the bones, e.g., skin, fat, and muscle. Using this basic X ray the surgeon can determine whether there is a problem, and what it is.

The results of the cephalogram are compared with the impressions that have been made of the patient's jaws and teeth. These models can be cut in various ways to simulate the contemplated surgery, and together with the X rays, allow the surgeon to determine what surgical steps are necessary in order to bring about facial harmony.

These studies of models and X rays are very important in order to minimize error. A surgeon can practice on the models any number of times, but there is usually only one chance to operate on a patient. The surgeon knows what he is going to do, precisely and mathematically, before he does it.

Poor relationships between the upper and lower jaws are the major cause of facial imbalance. The nose and lips may well in turn be affected by these. The profile can also be affected by the relation-

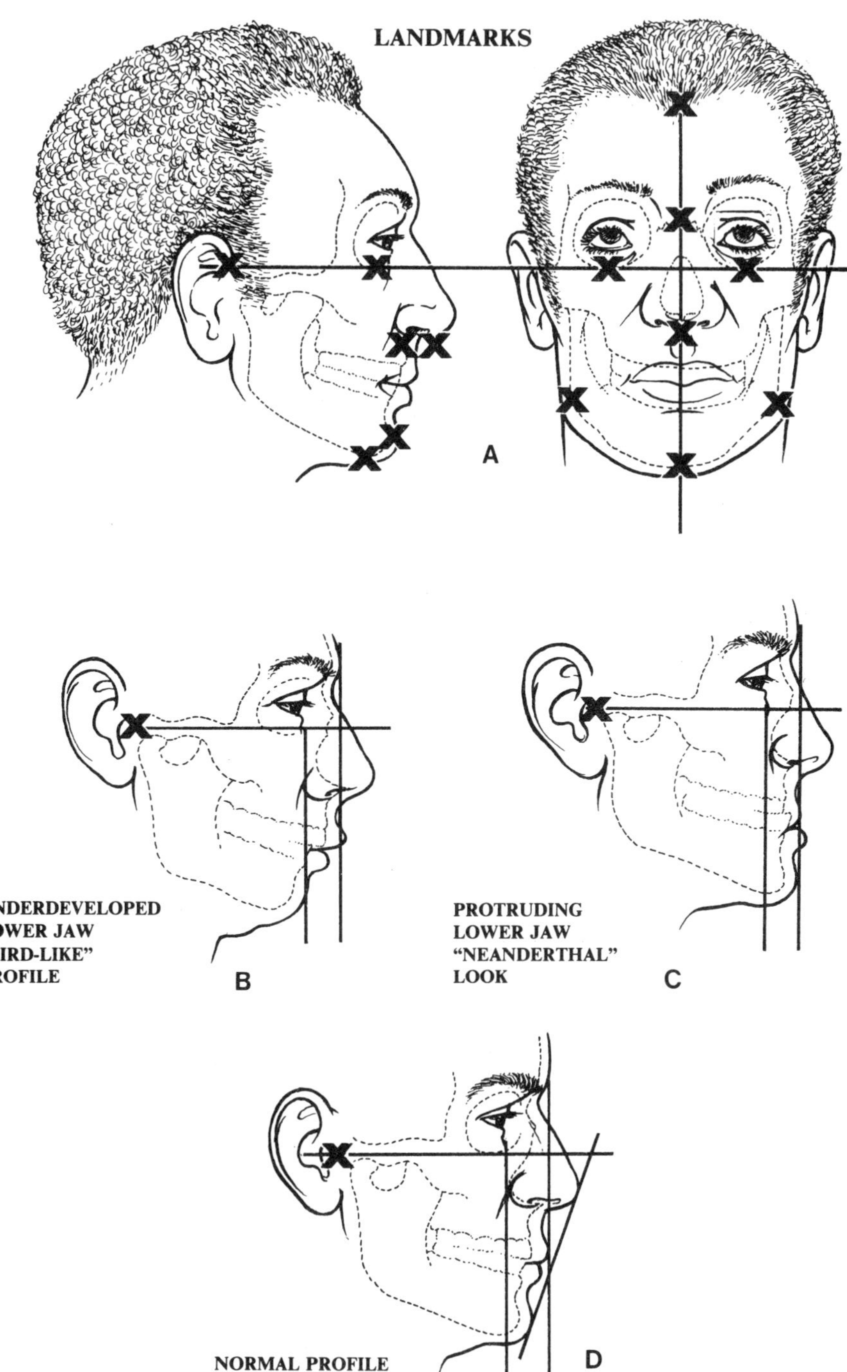

A. Critical anatomic landmarks used to study proposed surgical procedures and movements

B. A variety of possible jaw positions

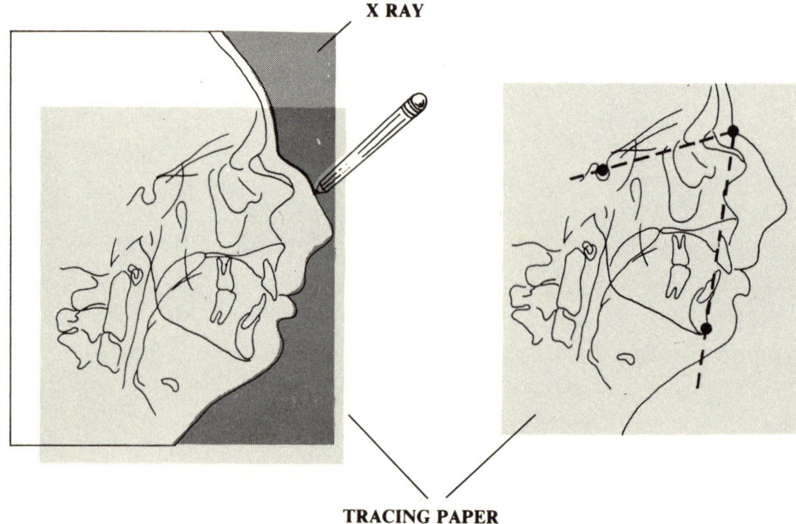

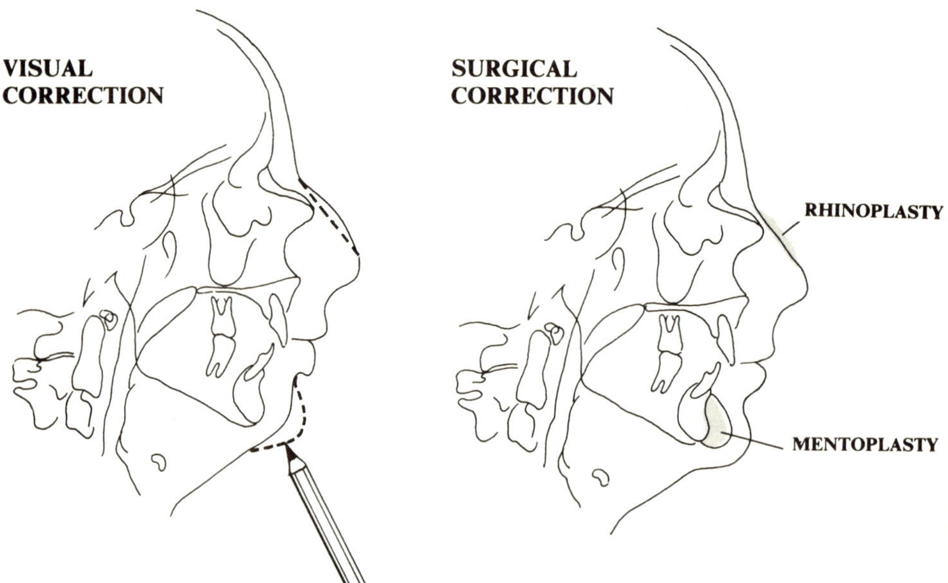

Cephalometrics—The Study of the Proposed Facial Corrections

A. An X-ray plate of the skull reveals the outline of the soft tissue (muscle, fat, skin) in contrast to the underlying bony structure.

B. A tracing paper copy of this is made. In this case, a large nose and receding chin are the problems.

C. The correction to be performed is outlined in pencil.

D. A rhinoplasty and chin augmentation correct the problem.

ship of the upper and lower teeth. In 1899, Dr. E. H. Angle classified the possible relationships of teeth of the upper and lower jaw into three classes:

Class 1—Normal profile
Class 2—Underdeveloped lower jaw, "birdlike" profile
Class 3—Protruding lower jaw, "Neanderthal type" look

Cephalometrics is a method of analysis. The skeletal (bony) and soft-tissue structures of the face are visualized on an X-ray plate, and having different densities they are easily differentiated from each other. Using predetermined points of reference, we can analyze the relationships of the various bony structures of the face to each other and to the overlying soft-tissue structures—lip, nose, etc. Certain norms have been worked out for each ethnic group and are utilized to determine what is to be done for a more harmonious appearance within that grouping.

Anthropologists and orthodontists have established certain landmarks on the facial skeleton that are used to follow growth patterns of the face, and to study the relationships of the upper and lower jaw. While the landmarks are the same—e.g., chin point, nasal bones, position of the orbital rim (the rim of the eye socket)—their relationship to each other, as well as the relationship of the jaws themselves, varies from the Caucasian to the Negroid to the Oriental groups.

Jaw deformities can occur within either the maxilla (upper jaw) or mandible (lower jaw). Several conditions can exist in both. The lower jaw can be either too far forward or backward.

If the lower jaw is too far forward, the term "mandibular prognathism" applies and is characterized by a so-called "lantern" jaw, giving the individual a Neanderthal type of look. The underdeveloped jaw can give a variety of appearances from a slightly weak chin to the more severe birdlike profile.

Similarly, there can be problems with the maxilla and its position in relationship to the mandible. These may result from failure of the upper jaw to develop, such as in cleft lip and cleft-palate deformities of birth. They can occur as a result of problems during the early facial development of the youngster, or from accidents. Defects range from minor facial growth disturbances, such as protrusion of the upper teeth and jaw, to more severe mid-facial lack of growth, resulting in the so-called "dish face" appearance.

CASE HISTORIES

Men who come to my office to discuss chin and jaw surgery give a variety of valid reasons for wanting the operation performed. One may complain, "My chin looks weak," while another may express his need for jaw surgery by saying "I can't chew properly," or "When I yawn, my jaw locks in an open position." There are other patients, however, who aren't even aware that chin surgery may be of help. Such a patient is Greg J.

A twenty-seven-year-old sheet metal worker, Greg came to my office to discuss having his nose shortened. I agreed that his nose was proportionally too long for his face. But I went a step further and suggested that he consider having his chin augmented. Greg was taken aback. I could tell he was thinking he was a candidate for a ripoff—two operations when one would do. He knew his nose needed reconstruction, but he thought the rest of him was fine.

We sat down and studied photographs of his face that I had ordered taken from many angles. It was the first time Greg truly saw each feature, rather than just a face dominated by a large nose. I pointed out that rhinoplasty would improve his looks considerably, but that bringing the chin forward by only a few millimeters would do even more for his appearance, as it would give better facial balance and symmetry.

The rhinoplasty and the chin augmentation operation were performed in my office surgical complex on the same day. The chin was augmented with a Silastic implant placed through a small incision inside his mouth. The combination of the two procedures resulted in a more harmonious appearance.

Another patient, Charles P., is a slightly built electrical engineer. Charles came to my office three years ago, at age twenty-four, because of a problem involving his bite. He was also concerned that the protrusion of his lower jaw and teeth gave him, he said, a "Neanderthal" look. His dentist, concerned with the bad bite and recurrent jaw dislocation, had referred him to me, believing that if the jaw were set back the chronic dislocations would be improved.

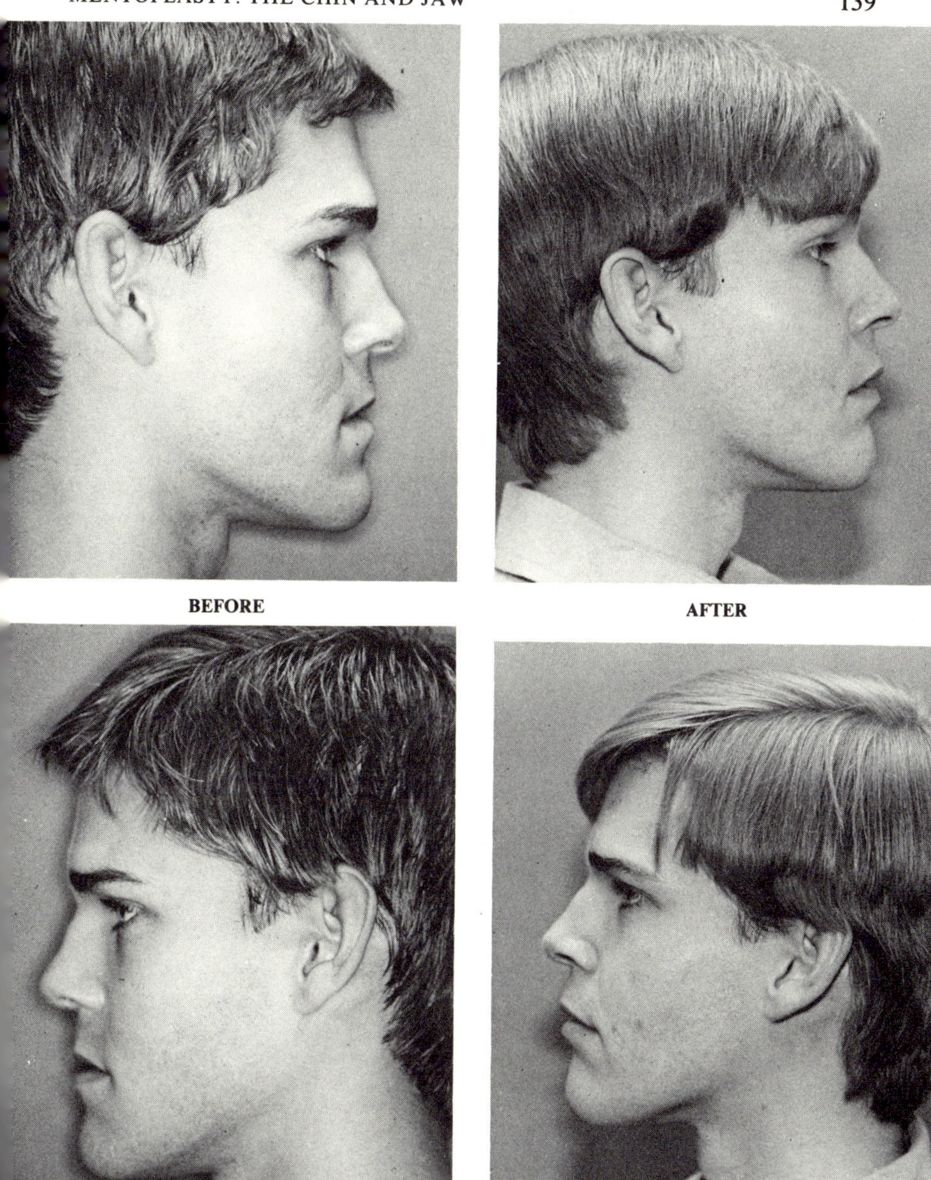

BEFORE AFTER

BEFORE AFTER

Protruding Jaw Correction

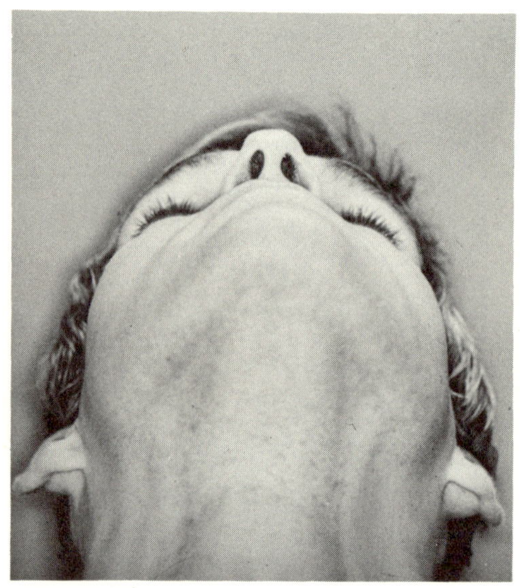

BEFORE

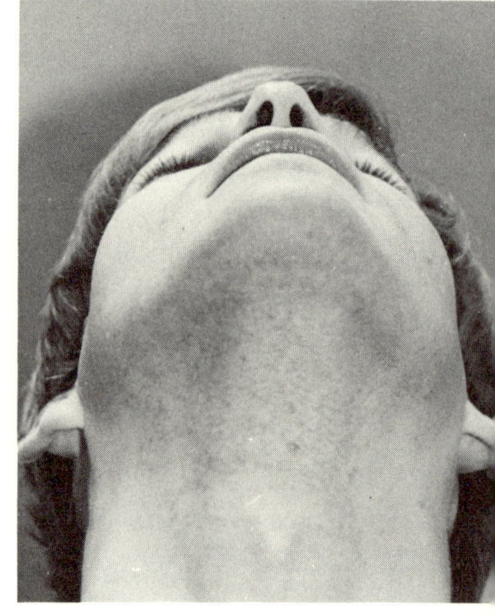

AFTER

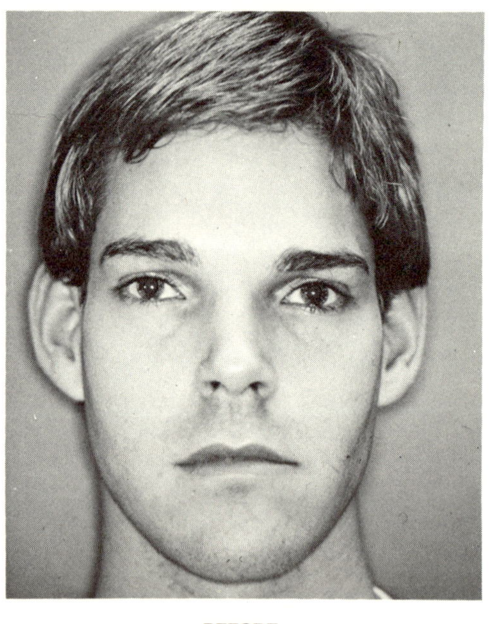

BEFORE

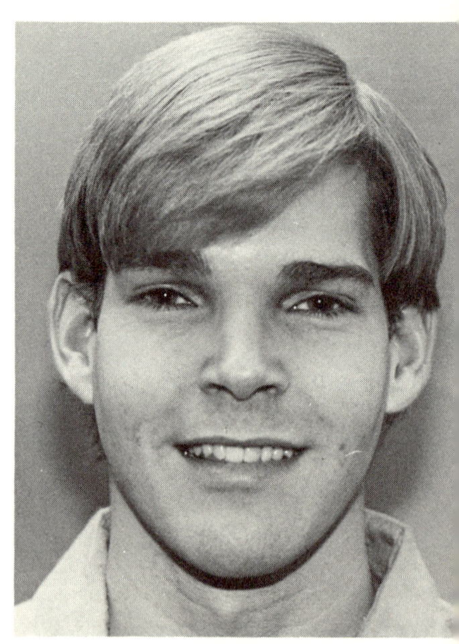

AFTER

However, I discovered that the overbite wasn't the only or even the main reason Charles needed work. His jaw would chronically dislocate if he yawned, or even opened his mouth too wide. When this happened Charles usually was able to put his fingers inside his mouth and pull the jaw down, forward, and then back into position. But whenever he was unable to correct it on his own, Charles would have to go to the hospital for injections into the masseter muscle (one of the major muscles that moves the jaw) so that it would relax. This would enable the doctors to then pull the jaw down and move it back to its normal position.

So Charles had problems—more problems than usual. First he had a cosmetic problem because of a prognathic, or "lantern," jaw; then he had a functional problem with his bite; and finally, a problem with a chronically dislocated jaw. After a series of X rays and much study of possible alternative methods of treatment it was determined that the jaw was too far forward but that the rest of his facial structures were in proportion.

Surgery was performed in the hospital. The jawbone was cut and allowed to slide back, thus shortening the protruding jaw. The bone fragments were wired together and arch bars were placed on the upper and lower teeth to immobilize the jaws. Since no jaw motion was possible after the operation, nourishment in the way of liquid food had to be sipped through a straw. Charles was in the hospital for five days, during which time the initial post-op swelling had decreased significantly. The arch bars remained on for about six weeks, to immobilize the jaws until they had healed solidly.

Have Charles's problems been solved? Cosmetically, the jaw is more acceptable. There is also a tremendous improvement in his bite—better dental occlusion will assure longer life for his teeth. And in the three years since surgery there has not been one instance of jaw dislocation. The only complaint is mine, and not a serious one at that. The last time I saw Charles he was sporting a full beard and mustache. I said, "Why hide your chin after all that work?" Charles said he was delighted with his new appearance, but just wanted a beard. He was pleased to wear one, I suppose, simply because he didn't *have* to hide behind one.

A Japanese-American patient was also sent to me by his dentist, in this case because of a severe underbite. Peter's lower jaw retruded so far back that it looked as if he had no chin at all. Cephalometric studies revealed that merely moving the jaw forward would not by itself give the desired result. An operation was performed to move the jaw containing the lower teeth forward, and a Silastic implant was inserted to make it even more prominent. Additionally, an operation was performed to take out the excess fat in Peter's neck to further improve his profile—we frequently need multiple procedures to get the final result.

SELF-EVALUATION

If you have severe malocclusion (abnormality in the coming together of teeth) that can't be readily corrected by conventional orthodontics, your dentist may be the one to recommend surgical realignment of the jaw. If your chin or jaw is not right for your face—say, it recedes and gives you a "weak" appearance—you don't have to have a dentist or anyone else tell you that you might consider having something done.

When you have a chin that needs augmentation, the only question to resolve is whether to have a Silastic implant or to have a part of the jaw itself moved forward. This is a matter for you to discuss with your surgeon. There are advantages to either method. You may discover, in fact, that your chin is all right, but that an overly long nose makes the chin appear inadequate.

In some situations, certain defects of the jaw can be camouflaged to a degree with a beard and mustache. But not every man is satisfied with cover-ups.

PROCEDURE

Before any jaw is realigned, the surgeon studies and restudies the models that have been made of the patient's jaws. The surgery itself is complex, for it involves cutting and moving bone, and so it is performed in a hospital. Plastic surgeons often utilize colleagues in dental and maxillo-facial surgery for a multidisciplinary approach.

The operation is performed under general anesthesia, with a tube passed through the nose into the trachea. The tube is usually placed through the nose rather than through the mouth because the surgeon needs as much room to work as possible. The fewer obstructions in the mouth, the better.

Most of the surgical work is done intra-orally so that there will be no visible scars. Special cheek retractors are used; they allow the surgeon to have the best view possible when he works in the small confines of the oral cavity. Specific instruments have been designed for the surgery, such as electric reciprocating saws with very fine blades. These saws enable the surgeons to cut the jawbone at various angles and in certain predetermined ways.

While all chin-jaw conditions require precise and often technically involved preoperative planning, I will briefly describe the basic surgical procedures to correct the most common deformities seen.

Microgenia, or Small Chin

Here, the cases most commonly encountered are those performed in conjunction with a rhinoplasty, where a minimal chin or jaw augmentation helps give the face a more harmonious appearance. The simplest method involves a soft silicone rubber implant placed directly on top of the bone and beneath the protection of the skin and fatty tissue of the chin. Problems can occasionally develop with this technique, particularly when the implant used is excessively large or is placed in a tight pocket with unyielding overlying skin. In some instances this can result in continued pressure on the underlying mandible, resultant bone loss, and even possible impingement on the roots of the teeth, ultimately requiring removal of the implant. Excessively tight skin can result in an implant's migration or slight shift. The result is contour abnormalities that require repositioning or replacement with a smaller implant.

There are two basic procedures that the plastic surgeon uses to augment a chin. One involves the insertion of a Silastic implant through a small incision inside the mouth. Because a foreign body is being inserted, there is always the potential risk of infection and the implant having to be temporarily removed; however, a new one can be put in later. An injury to the chin could also cause problems for the implant; it may shift out of place or even start to extrude as the result of trauma. Despite such possible complications, this technique is widely accepted as a means of minimal jaw augmentation.

SIMPLE BONE AUGMENTATION

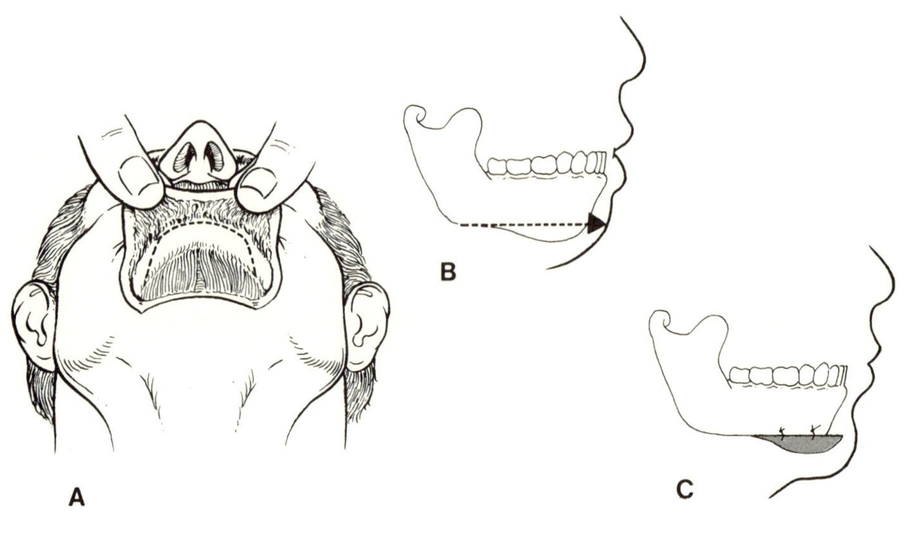

COMPLEX BONE AUGMENTATION

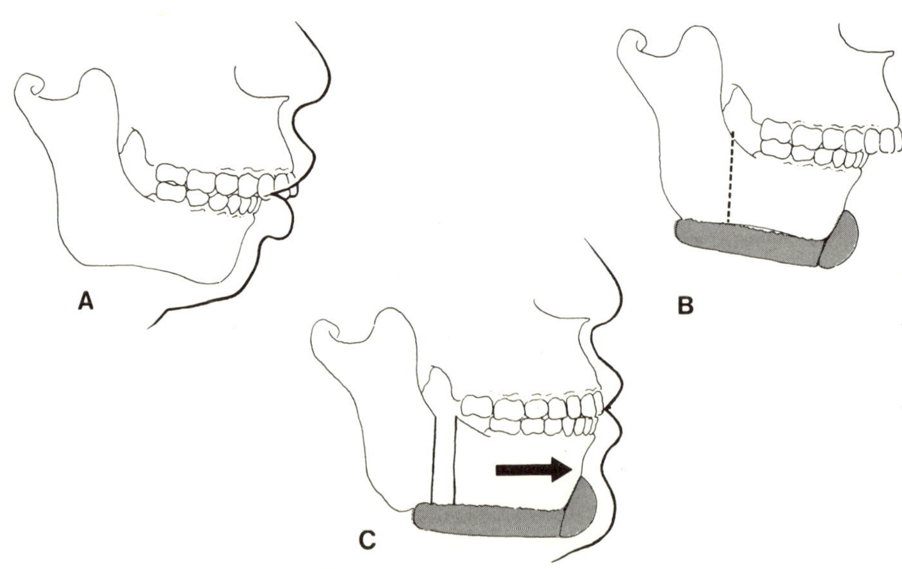

The other technique involves the actual repositioning of the jaw—forward, backward, even up or down. It is a slightly more complicated operation, but still considered safe. Here, the surgeon makes an incision inside the mouth. He then pulls the lower lip down and exposes the jawbone—a so-called "de-gloving" maneuver. With an oscillating saw he cuts across the lower portion of the jaw so that it can be pulled forward. The cut is made below the roots of the teeth to prevent injury to them. The lower teeth maintain their "bite" relationship with the upper teeth. The point of the chin is merely being augmented or advanced by use of the available bone.

The lower portion of the mandible, separated from the part of the jaw that contains the teeth, is brought forward and wired into position; two or three fine wires are used to fix the bone and hold it in its new forward position. It takes four to six weeks for the bones to heal. What has been accomplished, in other words, is a fracturing of the bone, creating a horizontal wedge, which is then advanced forward and wired into position. The wires usually remain permanently and cause no problems. This more permanent augmentation of the chin is called a horizontal advancement osteotomy. This surgical technique avoids the problem of shifting and possible extrusion of the soft silicone implant. To achieve facial harmony, more severe cases of small chin or jaw may require the onlay of bone or Silastic in addition to the advancement of the jaw.

Opposite page: Chin and Jaw Surgery (Mentoplasty)

Simple Bony Augmentation:

A. The incision is made inside the mouth, along the dotted line.

B. The dotted line shows the horizontal wedge of bone which is to be cut and moved forward.

C. The bony cuts have been made. The bone is slid forward and wired in place, resulting in profile augmentation

Complex Bony Augmentation:

A. The diagram shows a severe jaw retrusion.

B. The lower jaw bone and its contained teeth is cut and moved forward. Further augmentation with bone lengthens the vertical height as well as giving forward jaw projection.

C. Final resultant profile augmentation.

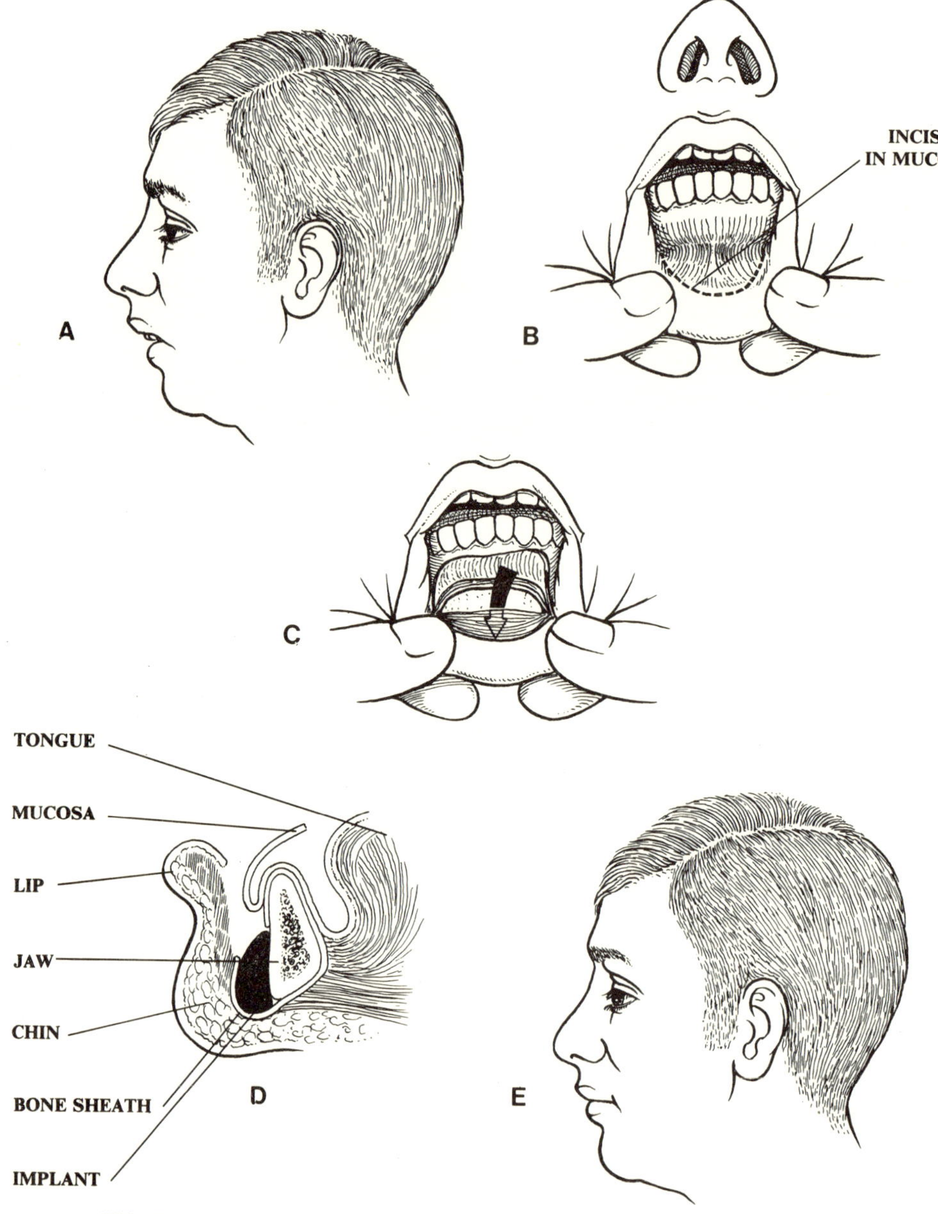

***Chin Implant* (*Mentoplasty*)**

A. Profile of a patient with a "weak" chin.

B. The lip is pulled down and the dotted line indicates the incision to be made inside the mouth.

C. The incision is made and the chin point is visualized.

D. A pocket has been created to receive the soft Silastic implant.

E. The final result shows the change in appearance.

The Prognathic or Forward Jaw

In addition to giving an imbalanced and often objectionable feature, the prognathic jaw is frequently accompanied by a poor dental condition. The normal maxillary or upper arch cannot make contact with the lower jaw. This results in an ineffective dental occlusional relationship; that is, the "bite" is bad. Correction can not only give a more pleasing facial appearance but improve the dental health of the individual. The incisions are usually intraoral and the jaw containing the teeth is moved backward.

Anterior Open Bite

This is a condition resulting in a variable degree of protruding upper teeth; it can be corrected by what is termed a segmental movement of the upper six anterior teeth. This set-back, or movement, may be accomplished by removal of the first premolar teeth on both sides, and segmental movement of the six anterior (front) teeth posteriorly (back) and inferiorly (down).

AFTER SURGERY

A patient can expect to be in the hospital for up to a week after jaw reconstruction. Because the bone has been moved and cut there is an inordinate amount of facial swelling; it takes several weeks for this swelling to go down, and about two months for the repositioned bones to heal. During this period splints are kept in place to immobilize the upper and lower jaws and fix them to each other.

With your jaws immobile, it's no surprise to find yourself on a liquid diet. There's no reason, however, why you shouldn't be getting the proper nourishment during this time. For the first few days after the operation you will be fed through a tube passed from the nose into the stomach. Soon afterwards, liquid nourishment can be given orally despite the teeth being wired.

If there has been a Silastic implant to augment your chin, this is usually a minor procedure that ordinarily doesn't require hospitalization. Extreme caution should be used to make sure that the new chin is not disturbed or jolted for a month or so after surgery. You

FORWARD JAW

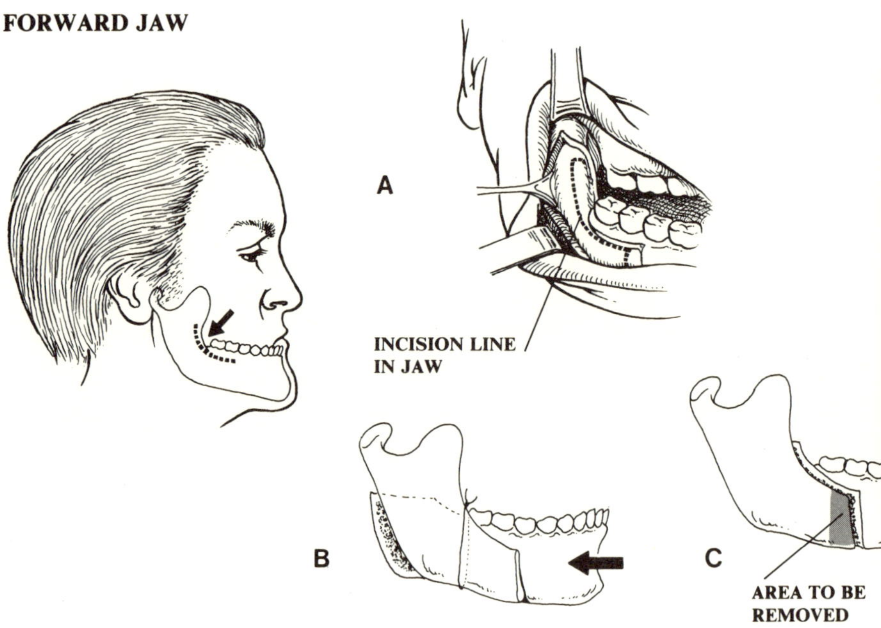

A. The incision for surgery is made inside the mouth, thus avoiding external scars.

B. The jaw is cut in the appropriate place and the forward segment containing the teeth is then slid backward.

C. The result of the correction.

"DISH-FACE"

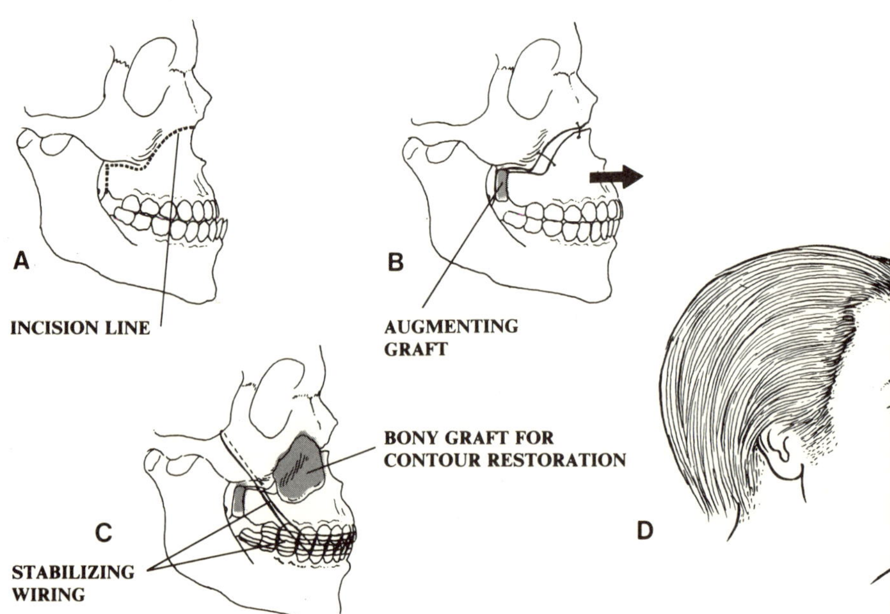

can, however, get to work within only a week or ten days. By then the swelling will have gone down significantly.

WHAT CAN GO WRONG

When a chin is augmented with a Silastic rubber implant, a foreign body has been introduced. If the chin is traumatized or severely bumped, the implant can be moved out of position and may have to be repositioned in a second operation. Replacement would also be a necessity if the implant is the source of an infection. Drainage may require removal of an implant, which usually can be reinserted at a later date, although complications associated with implants are infrequent.

The procedure of moving the jaw forward or backward is a more major and complex procedure, so there is a possibility of more complications. Because bones have been cut and repositioned there will be a great deal of swelling and some black and blue discoloration. These problems, however, resolve themselves within a relatively brief period of time, about two or three weeks. There have been some rare occasions of bone infection after surgery, but such infection is treatable with antibiotics.

WHAT YOU CAN EXPECT

Your expectations should depend on the type of surgery performed. A chin augmentation operation, for example, can improve your looks in several ways. Not only does the chin gain new prominence but the harmony of the face is improved. The same applies when the jaw is made less prominent.

"Dish-Face"

A. The outline of the cuts in the upper jaw and maxilla necessary for the correction.

B. The upper segment moved forward. A bone block is used to stabilize and keep it forward.

C. The teeth are wired and a bone graft added for further contouring and facial projection.

D. The resulting profile.

TEN

Rhytidectomy: The Total Face-Lift

THE FACE-LIFT is not a new process. Its popularity, however, has reached tremendous proportions only within the last ten or fifteen years. Acceptance by men in all walks of life has not only been stimulated by the knowledge that a variety of celebrities—show business personalities and politicians—have had face-lifts, but the positive experiences of friends and co-workers have helped make the art of looking good far more popular. No longer is it considered effeminate to care for one's appearance.

In the beginning, those who chose to have a rhytidectomy, or, as it is popularly called, the face-lift, were almost exclusively women. Considered to be a cosmetic luxury and beautification device available only to the rich and famous, the procedure was kept ultra secret, something to be talked about as little as possible and then only in hushed tones behind drawing-room doors.

Although we're not quite certain just when the first rhytidectomy was performed, it was in the early 1900s that the technique was employed successfully and with some regularity, both here and in Europe. However, only in the past decade has there been a significant shift among those choosing to have face-lifts: about 30 percent of the patients who now come to me are men.

The Signs of Aging

Rare is the man who reaches the age of fifty without noticing and feeling some of the subtle signs of the natural aging process: less muscular strength, poorer vision, more graying hairs or no hair at all. Most men find that the effects of their advancing years become increasingly apparent. Scientists still have not found a way to reverse this aging process. Perhaps later we will not only find a way to

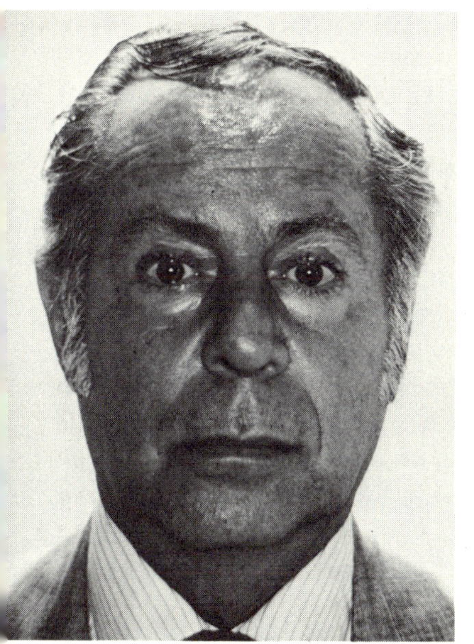

BEFORE

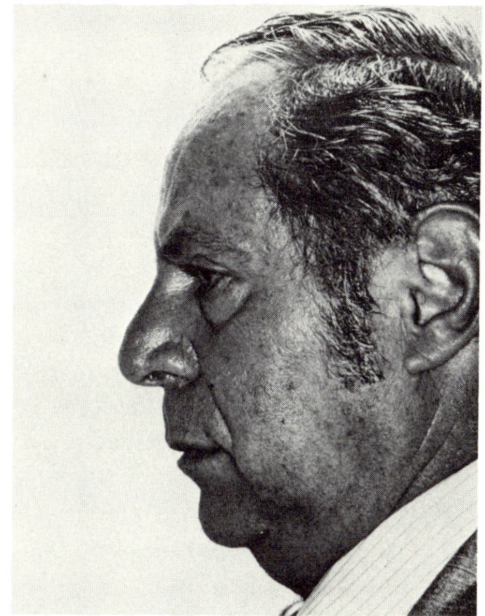

BEFORE

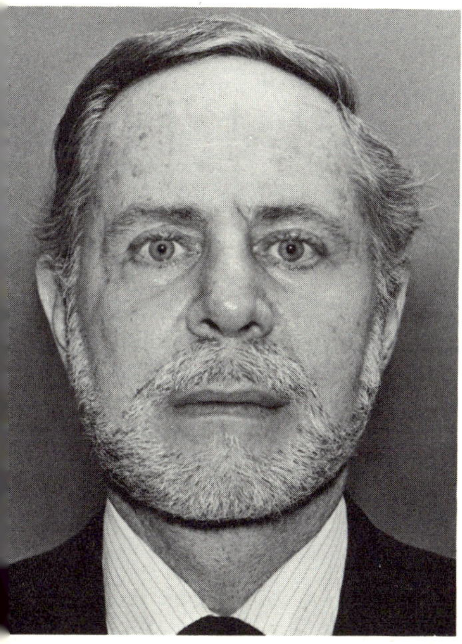

AFTER

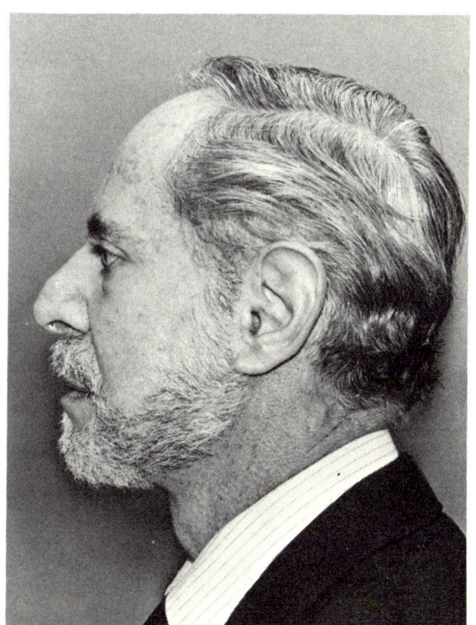

AFTER

A dramatic example of the benefits of a total face-lift. The man's appearance is more youthful and his expression more vital and dynamic. Growing a beard really topped off his new look.

prolong the human life-span significantly, but also to modify advancing symptoms of age. It is with these more visible signals that we're concerned with here—lined and wrinkled skin, sagging of jowls, less elasticity—the signs that most frequently distress a man when he looks into the mirror. For all too often, as a man ages, he feels younger than he looks.

Many of the first signs of aging appear in the skin, an early indicator of what is going on internally. For the skin is living matter that breathes and protects our body. What causes its cellular structure to go through the aging process is still mostly theory, but it is known that one reason for the loss of skin tone is alterations in the structure and quantity of collagen, a gelatinous protein and the chief component of the connective tissue and organic substance of both skin and cartilage. Comparable changes in elastin—the chief constituent of elastic fibers that make up the connective tissue elements—make the skin more flabby.

Although no cell or tissue is unaffected by age, it is the collagen, representing 75 percent of the skin's composition, that goes through structural changes resulting in thinner, less resilient skin. Collagen is a major structural component of the skin. It is a molecule and consists of a three-coil polypeptide (chain) made of amino acids (protein). Collagen is continually made or synthesized. It is also being degraded, or broken down, in an ongoing process. Its metabolic activity continues throughout life, but decreases with aging. Fibers become progressively thicker until age twenty, with minimal increases thereafter.

Other changes take place with age. They include thinning and fewer pigment-containing granules of the epidermis. Within the dermis, the collagen becomes more resistant or less resilient. There is also a decrease of elastic fibers. These same changes within the collagen may also account for both the atrophy of bone structure and certain diseases associated with the arteries—two problems of advancing age. Such changes affect both sexes equally. The question of who ages faster, a man or a woman, has far more to do with genetic makeup than with masculinity and femininity.

When the skin loses its elasticity, it produces some of the more visible signs of aging familiar to all of us. These include subtle changes in skin texture, more open pores in some cases, wrinkles or

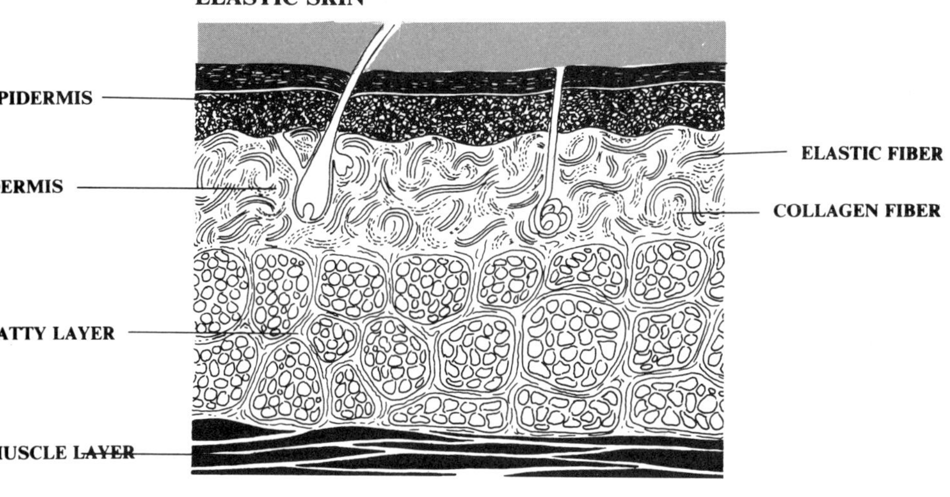

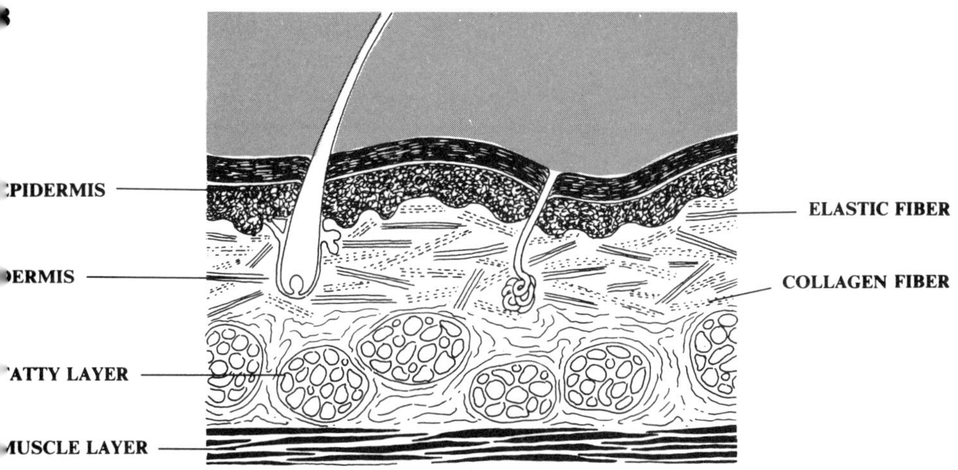

Skin Change (Rhytidectomy)

A. The elastic and supple skin of a young adult showing an abundance of elastic and collagen fibers in the dermal layer and a substantial fatty layer.

B. Loss of elasticity with advancing age. Notice the decrease of the elastic and collagen fibers as well as the decrease of the fatty layer.

fine lines that form with increasing ease, and, finally, less flexibility as the skin no longer seems to fit the structure beneath it and begins to sag or fold indiscriminately. That's when we notice the jowls, bags, deep furrows, and creases that mark the ravages of time and the forces of gravity on the face.

Of course, all of these factors affect individuals at different times and in different degrees. Some men accept pouches and sags at age fifty that others would seek to remove at forty. Often, an individual's emotional response to how he looks determines whether or not he will decide to have cosmetic surgery, and when he will have it.

When a man questions why he may seem to age faster than another, I cannot give him an adequate answer. Actually, many factors are responsible for the rate and acceleration of aging. They include mental and physical trauma, heredity and the care we give—or don't give—ourselves. If you don't exercise enough, if you eat and drink the wrong foods, if you smoke excessively, and if your lifestyle is unnecessarily stressful, you may well become old before your time and look it.

The sun is also a great cause of aging. As the sun causes the skin to lose its moisture, wrinkles occur. Excessive exposure to sunlight is inadvisable for all, but especially to any individual of light complexion or with a tendency toward dry skin. Sudden weight loss, too, may cause premature wrinkles and excess skin that no longer has the elasticity and resilience to fit the underlying bone structure; for as the skin deteriorates, there is frequently a loss of muscle tone along with it.

Crisis situations also create new needs. For those men who separate or divorce, who are seeking new social lives and relationships, or for those who feel that they can't compete in the job market, there may be special concern about their appearance. If you have ever thought, "If only I were ten years younger, or *looked* ten years younger . . ." then perhaps you too have considered cosmetic surgery of the face.

Fortunately, a man who wants to improve his looks and turn the clock back can often do so, for there have been remarkable advances in both the theories and techniques of plastic surgery. No longer is embarrassment a factor, and as a result more and more men are taking advantage of the plastic surgeon's skills. As I've mentioned, in my practice it is no longer unusual for me to find that nearly 30 percent of the consultations scheduled in a week are men who are seriously considering a face-lift. What is more, many are getting them.

CASE HISTORIES

Most if not all men who contemplate a face-lift want to look younger. And there's no doubt that a face-lift can do just that. One seventy-one-year-old patient of mine is proof. About two weeks after Martin R. had his face-lift he had an appointment with me for a checkup. He had gone into the subway and expected to use the half-price pass that is given out in New York to those sixty-five years of age and over. The subway toll booth attendant asked him to fish out his identification and prove he was sixty-five, which Martin did with pleasure. Before surgery, the subway attendants would just gaze at his face, know that he was over sixty-five, and let him pass.

By the way, the reason Martin had come to see me in the first place was that his seventeen-year-old daughter from a second marriage was about to graduate from high school. He simply didn't want everyone at the commencement ceremony to assume that his daughter was his granddaughter. In addition, he was in the catering business in Florida, and mentioned that looking much younger than his calendar years wouldn't hurt business.

Some men come to consult with me about a face-lift at the first signs of skin laxity. John H., a forty-seven-year-old insurance company executive, wanted the operation, although at first I said there didn't seem to me to be a need, that, in fact, he looked fine for his age. John insisted it would help. Eventually, I agreed to perform the operation although I was a bit skeptical. As it turned out, I was able to remove more skin than I had first thought possible and there was a definite improvement in John's appearance; he achieved a very youthful look.

For some men who come for the rhytidectomy there is no doubt at all that they will profit from it. One fifty-two-year-old patient who comes to mind looked like "Plastic Man" in the Dick Tracy comic strip. Don C.'s skin was loose and flabby and his neck was sagging. He probably should have had the operation performed years before, for from the quality of his skin and its elasticity it was

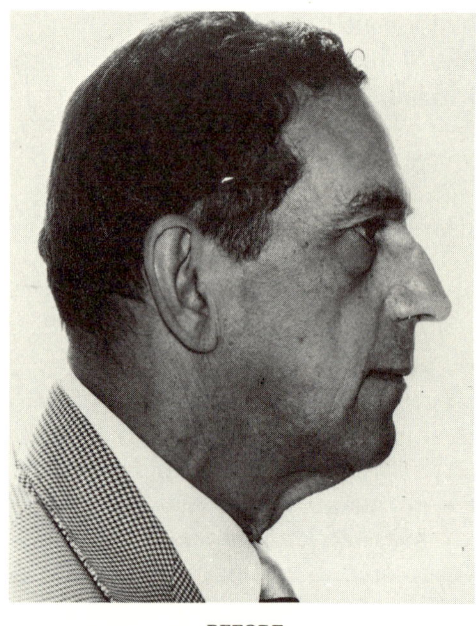

BEFORE

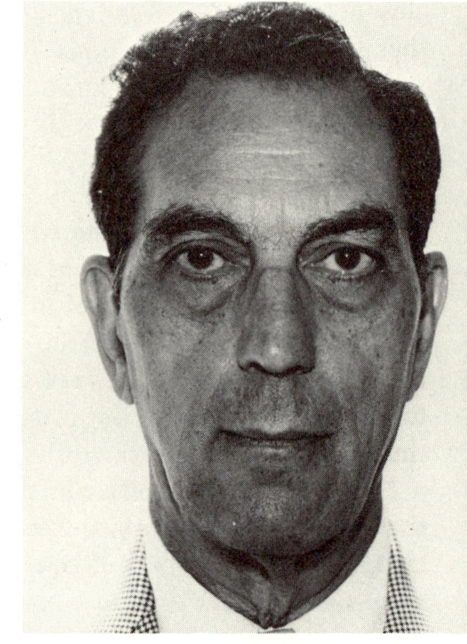

BEFORE

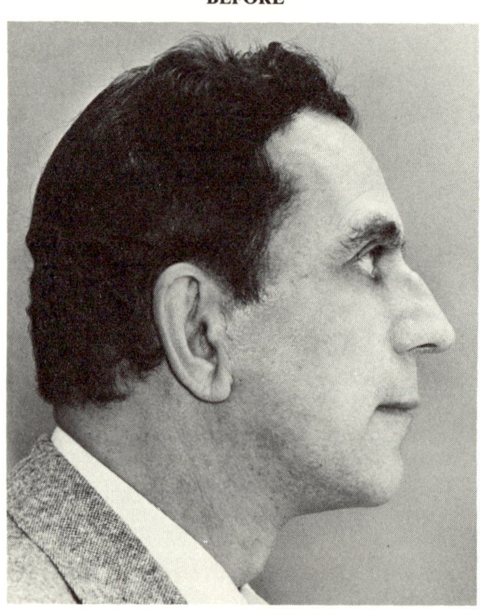

AFTER

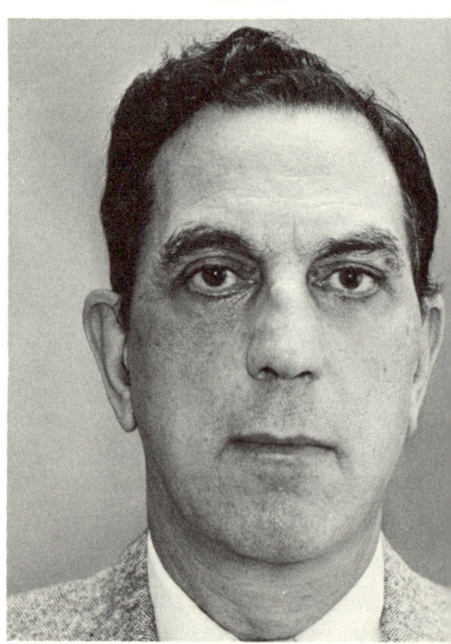

AFTER

The Total Face-Lift (Rhytidectomy)—Before and After

clear that it had aged very rapidly. He would have benefited from the results of the face-lift even sooner.

A total face-lift does not require a long recuperative period, important to a man with limited time to spare. Within a week or ten days a man will be sufficiently recovered and can resume most of his normal activities. One patient of mine had a face-lift and within two weeks embarked on a trip to Russia and the Scandinavian countries. He had let his hair grow long and combed it to conceal the healing incisions. I'm sure no one could tell that he had had any surgery performed. While total baldness may make concealing the incisions difficult, a toupee could adequately hide them, but most men are not totally bald and the existing hair, though sparse, will usually cover the incision sites.

Many men have face-lifts because they want to look better for themselves but quite often it is a work-related reason that brings them to my office. For instance, I recently operated on a seventy-year-old landscape designer. Peter V. had retired at the age of sixty, but with inflation and the increasing cost of living, he discovered that he was getting into a financial bind and needed extra income. He decided to get back into the job market, and while he looked considerably younger than his seventy years, he felt that an even more youthful appearance would help him. After I performed a complete face-lift, along with eyelid surgery, Peter was hired by a landscape architectural firm. He is now working part time and gaining the extra income he desired.

SELF-EVALUATION

If you are considering a face-lift, you can find out if you're a candidate simply by looking into the mirror and noting the signs you see of aging. Deepening of the lines and creases of the face, sagginess about the jawline, and an excess amount of skin on the neck are probably the most commonplace complaints of the man seeking surgery.

You can contemplate the results of a face-lift simply by taking the tips of your fingers of both hands and placing them on your face and then giving a gentle upward push. This simple test will, to a certain degree, re-create the improvement that can be gained through plastic surgery. It is by no means a perfect measure of the end result, but it will give you an idea of what can be done.

The best candidate for a face-lift is a male in good health in his late forties through fifties; in most cases this type of patient gets the best results because his skin still retains much of its tone, and its elasticity hasn't been greatly diminished. The results can be quite remarkable.

Patients in their sixties and seventies will still see a considerable improvement but the face-lift will not last as long. This is because at that time of life, the skin has begun to deteriorate, the elastic fibers have begun to stretch, and their number is decreasing. This doesn't mean that the procedure shouldn't be performed on an older man, only that he should realize that the results may be less striking because of his age. Often a secondary procedure may be elected if there is excess skin that can still be removed.

BEFORE SURGERY

The Consultation

Assuming good physical health and a mature state of mind, most men who visit a plastic surgeon generally are good candidates for the operation. It has been my experience that a man usually comes to my office after having already given a great deal of thought to what he wants to accomplish. The consultation generally confirms his prior ideas.

When you are consulting with a surgeon, be sure to ask and discuss anything that is on your mind; don't feel that any of your questions are frivolous or unnecessary. The physician, of course, will want to know why you came to him and probably will hand you a mirror so you can point out exactly what is bothering you. He will then be able to tell you which of those problems are correctible.

During the initial interview your doctor will obtain information on the general condition of your health, including a history of allergies and any reactions to drugs. Certain medications, for example, could determine the anesthesia and type of dosage to be used. Your doctor will most certainly want to take into account whether you have hypertension or diabetes. It may be necessary to get clearance from another doctor who is treating you before the surgery is performed.

I have operated on many patients with medical problems, including several men who have had pacemakers implanted to correct cardiac irregularities. Assuming medical clearance has been obtained, very few health problems preclude the possibility of plastic surgery.

Preparation

One basic decision that has to be made—by doctor and patient—is where the surgery should be performed. A patient may choose the hospital for a variety of reasons; however, since most insurance policies specifically exclude cosmetic surgery and because of the ever increasing cost of hospitalization, more and more patients are choosing to have the surgery performed on an outpatient basis. Many surgeons have complete facilities for surgery in their office complexes—which are also equipped for the immediate postoperative recovery phase.

As an outpatient you generally arrive at the doctor's office about an hour before surgery. If, however, the surgery is performed in a hospital, you will be admitted either the night before or the morning of the surgery.

No matter where the operation is to be performed, you will probably be given an injection containing a sedative, usually about an hour before the procedure. This will adequately sedate you, freeing you from anxiety, yet allow you to be conscious so that you can respond to directions. In the operating room, or a room adjacent to it, your face will be prepared for surgery. Usually a minimal amount of hair is shaved, and only at the incision site. Surrounding hair may be braided with a rubber band or held out of the way with petroleum jelly. An attempt is made to leave as much hair as possible so that long hairs can cover the incision site while the healing occurs. You will be able to return to work and public life only a couple of weeks after the surgery, and in some cases even sooner.

Most surgeons use a local anesthesia with a blood vessel constrictor such as epinephrine (adrenalin). This allows the blood vesels under the skin to contract, and thus minimizes bleeding. The procedure can also be performed under general anesthesia, but the incidence of complications is even lower from local anesthesia.

Local anesthesia eliminates the need for a tube to be placed in the trachea, which would be necessary when administering general anesthesia. For one thing, it's easier for the surgeon to work without a tube in the operative field. Also, the placement of the tube in the trachea can cause some postoperative discomfort. Most patients with adequate preoperative sedation followed by local anesthesia are comfortable, and just drowsy enough not to mind being awake during the procedure. The mere thought of general anesthesia frightens many patients and if it can be avoided, so much the better.

Before the operation, an antiseptic solution—usually an iodine soap compound or pHisoHex soap—is applied on the facial and hair area. The operative site is then draped with sterile sheets and towels. The surgeon now outlines the area of the incision and injects it with a local anesthesia solution; after about five minutes the blood vessels have constricted, minimizing bleeding. The anesthetic has taken effect and the procedure begins.

THE PROCEDURE

The surgical procedure consists of incisions placed in the hairline and above the ear, as well as in front of the ear and behind the ear. The skin is elevated through these incisions and separated from the underlying muscles and bones of the face. It is then pulled upward and backward, with the excess skin removed and the new skin edge sutured to the incisions in the areas around the ear and in the hairline. The actual operation generally takes from two to four hours, depending on how much work is done; it can be combined with an eyelid operation as well.

A newly developed surgical technique enables the removal of fat around the neck area. A small incision is made under the chin—right under the prominence of the jawbone in an area which when healed is inconspicuous and well worth the improvement gained. The surgeon is able to lift the skin away and look right into the resultant tunnel. He is thus able to cut away accumulations of fat that couldn't be reached, or even observed, from the incision by the ear and hairline. Fat from the entire neck can be removed through this new procedure. Results have been excellent.

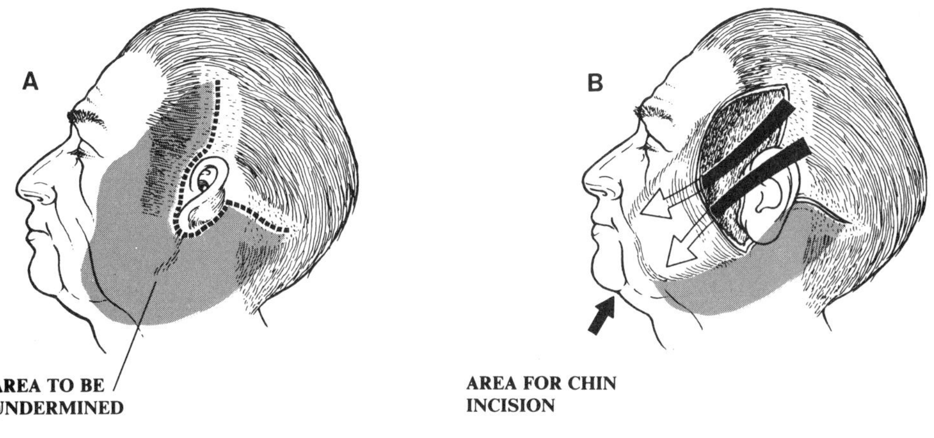

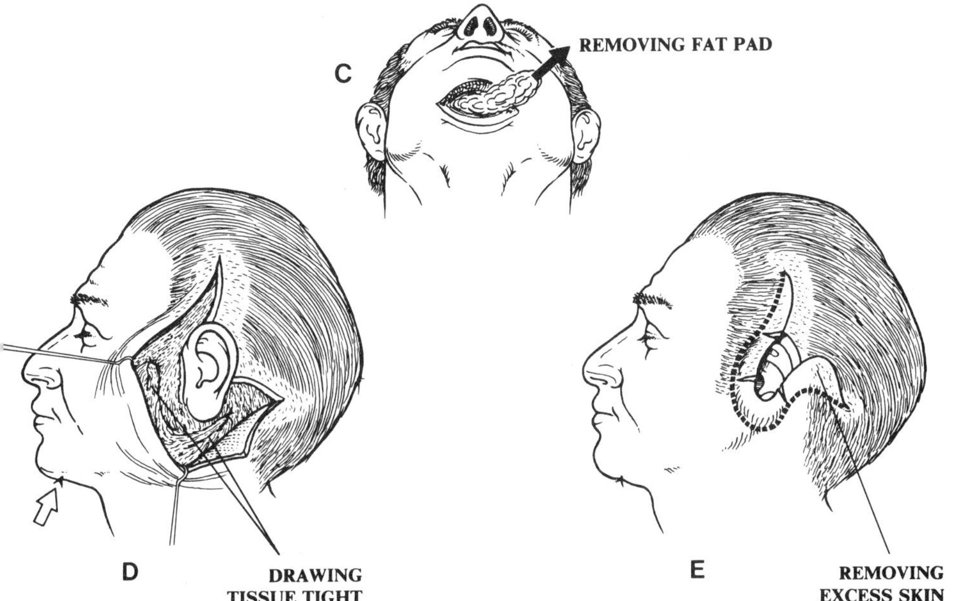

The Total Face-Lift (Rhytidectomy)

A. The standard incision for the male face-lift.

B. The area and extent of the undermining of the facial skin.

C. The submental (under the chin) incision which is used to remove fat in the neck area.

D. Sutures are used to firm up the deeper tissue layers beneath the skin.

E. The excess skin beyond the dotted line will be removed.

The small amount of bleeding that persists despite the blood-vessel constricting drugs is controlled by electrocautery. The surgeon usually tightens up the lax tissues of the face with sutures. This seems to give a better result, for it is these tissues that sag and create both jowls and drooping in the corners of the mouth. Finally, a drain is usually placed beneath the skin to allow for the collection of any tissue fluid or blood that occurs in the first twenty-four to forty-eight hours. The skin is then drawn superiorly and posteriorly and the excess removed; anchoring sutures are placed in critical positions around the incision site. The wound is usually closed with a fine suture material placed immediately below the skin and avoiding the conspicuous crosshatching effect formerly seen in older surgical techniques. The subcuticular stitch, or suture under the skin, leaves the most inconspicuous scar and is one of the hallmarks of a plastic surgical closure.

AFTER SURGERY

Not much discomfort is experienced, certainly no more than can be relieved by a mild pain-killing analgesic and possibly some sedation for a comfortable sleep; your surgeon will prescribe these for you. You can eat or drink anything you want, but I usually prescribe a soft diet, one that doesn't require extensive chewing. I also suggest that a patient keep his head elevated and that he prop himself up with at least two or three pillows when sleeping. This helps reduce postoperative swelling.

Your physician will usually be seeing you twenty-four to forty-eight hours after the operation, at which time he will remove the dressings, inspect the wounds, and check the drains and probably remove them. A less cumbersome dressing probably will be applied for the next twenty-four to forty-eight hours. After approximately seventy-two hours, all the dressings are usually removed. The anchor sutures are generally removed in four or five days and the remaining in about seven to ten days. I usually recommend that the patient use a mild shampoo several days after surgery to remove any prepping solution and any blood that might remain on the hair as a result of the surgery.

Most patients, secure in their appearance, return to work at the end of one or two weeks. Three weeks, however, is a safer interval, because while the wounds have usually all closed, some small areas may not have completely healed at the end of two weeks, and bruising may be evident as well. Nevertheless, there are some men who choose to return to work quite soon after surgery. It's an individual choice, based on individual needs.

I suggest you allow your hair to grow longer than usual before the operation because the extra hair will help camouflage the incision scar until it fades. When sideburns are in fashion, a longer sideburn might be elected. As far as the swelling itself is concerned, it will take several weeks before most of it is gone, and also for the operative site to lose some of that tight feeling.

WHAT CAN GO WRONG

As with any surgical procedure, complications can occur, and you should be aware of them. For example, the accumulation of small pockets of blood beneath the skin flaps is not too uncommon, occuring in a small percentage of cases. Surgery on a man requires a slightly deeper plane of dissection than necessary for a woman, in order to preserve the hair follicles, which are at a deeper level. There is therefore more bleeding and potential accumulation of blood with men. During the operation itself the surgeon will pay great attention to controlling bleeding. Postoperatively, in about 2 percent of cases, some blood will accumulate under the skin. Your surgeon will probably use a syringe to remove the blood pockets should they occur; larger accumulations may require a small incision or puncture of the skin to expel the coagulated blood. Blood pockets usually are noted within the first twenty-four to forty-eight hours after surgery, but they may not be noticed until several days later when the swelling comes down. These blood accumulations are easily taken care of and do not interfere significantly with the end result of the surgery. Nevertheless, the area where they occur may be slightly firm for an extended period of time.

Infection is rare, but if it does occur antibiotic treatment should resolve the problem. Superficial skin loss may occur occasionally in the area behind the ear. These areas heal without incident. Larger and more serious loss of skin is quite unusual.

A more alarming situation is temporary muscle weakness. This may occur because of the work being done in the proximity of the nerve that supplies movement to the eyebrow, and to the nerve that moves the lower lip muscles. These complications, however, are rare, and when they do occur, the weakness around the eyebrow and lower lip is usually temporary. This infirmity is usually due to the pull on the nerve, or to a direct injection into the nerve itself at the time when the anesthetic solution is given.

A more common occurrence, not to be considered a real complication, because it occurs in almost all patients and is then resolved, is a decrease in sensations in the facial area as well as the ear itself. Patients often say their ears don't feel as if they are their own. This strange sensation always normalizes. Other aftereffects that also resolve themselves are swelling and any black-and-blue marks.

WHAT YOU CAN EXPECT

In today's society the man with the ideal face has a nose that is in proportion with the rest of his face, a good jawline, and a long neck. If you don't have these attributes, a face-lift won't give them to you. When the surgeon drapes back your skin, he can only do over the face that you had before.

Face-lift surgery will not erase the first lines around the upper and lower lip, nor will it remove the vertical furrows above the nose—the frown lines. Neither is the operation meant to remove completely the normal nasolabial folds (lines from the nose to the corner of the mouth). In these cases, there are ancillary procedures that can further rejuvenate the face, like skin planing (dermabrasion) or chemical peeling, both of which are discussed elsewhere in this book.

There are men, generally those in their late sixties and older, who may be candidates for a second face-lift a few months after their first. This does not mean that the first one was unsuccessful. During the first procedure, skin is pulled up as tightly as possible and approximately an inch of skin removed from each side. If it were stretched any tighter, there might be some loss of blood supply to the area, resulting in skin loss and a wider scar formation. If a man is sixty or older when he first has a face-lift, there could be some relaxation of the skin, which is why a second operation might be beneficial. However, the skin will never sag to the degree it did before the first procedure, and he may well be enough improved in appearance not to want a second operation. But there are some men who have skin with such laxity that they decide to return to the surgeon within a year to obtain an even more spectacular result.

The younger man who has a face-lift ordinarily wouldn't need a secondary procedure right away; his skin is still quite firm. But there is bound to be a gradual deterioration as the aging process continues through the years, and so a second face-life may be desirable, the timing of it generally dependent on the individual's age. A man in his late forties or early fifties who has a face-lift probably won't need another for as long as seven to ten years.

Knowing what you can't expect from an operation is as important as knowing what you can expect. Plastic surgery, and particularly a face-lift, can be the beginning of a new and exciting stage in your life, but there is the danger that your expectations about the changes it will create in your lifestyle will be unrealistic. In that event you might become more discouraged, angry, and frustrated when things don't turn out according to your plans. If you have made a successful face-lift the basis of a whole new way of life or a means to achieving major goals, then you may well be doomed to disappointment. A new face will not give you a new life.

While plastic surgeons are not psychiatrists who treat deep-seated neuroses, we are all aware of some of the potential problems with those patients who seek surgery for nonrealistic reasons. During the initial consultations, these areas should be probed in detail by both you and your physician.

The end goal should be fully understood by both you and your doctor. Unrealistic expectations on your part can undermine an otherwise technically good result. If, for example, you cannot accept the inevitable fact of aging, you may be disappointed with the face-lift results. Surgery isn't the panacea for every patient's problems. You should thoroughly and honestly examine your motives in seeking any cosmetic reconstruction so that you will have an honest visualization of what you can truly derive from the expense, time, and commitment involved.

ELEVEN

Body Sculpturing and Contouring

MANY PEOPLE think of body contouring—or what is more popularly referred to as body sculpturing—as a surgical procedure performed mainly on women. In the past, women found a variety of reasons to be displeased with their silhouettes, and sought cosmetic changes: re-shaping because of extremes in weight loss and gain after crash dieting, or because of stretching of the abdomen and breasts during pregnancy. Often, new mothers return to their pre-pregnancy weight only to find that their abdomens still sag or their breasts have become pendulous. Breast reconstructions are performed after mastectomies, and surgery is often done to correct assymetrical breasts and to increase or decrease the size of breasts.

Today, however, men, too, choose to have plastic surgery performed on their abdomens and breasts, although their numbers are considerably smaller than those of women electing to have the same procedures. As a result of massive weight loss within a relatively brief time, some men find they are left with loose and flabby skin—hanging apronlike from the abdominal wall and extending over the thighs—that neither exercise nor diet will firm up or remove. I have seen many males, particularly adolescents, who have had tremendous weight problems. Although they resolved their obesity through diet, they ended up with a new problem: the skin, distended by the massive weight gain, became stretched beyond normal limits and could not return to its original state.

Abdominal lipectomy is actually a process whereby the skin that has lost its resilience is removed. An incision is usually made across the lower part of the abdomen, through the pubic hair line approximately four to six inches below the navel, enough to be hidden by bathing trunks. The skin is lifted up and away. A strip of skin is then removed, usually eighteen to twenty-four inches long and about six or eight inches high. The strip encompasses almost the entire amount of abdominal skin below the navel. After this, the abdominal skin above the navel is separated from the underlying muscle tissues and pulled down to replace the skin that has been removed. The cut edges are then sutured.

However, the navel is still attached to the muscles and tissue of the abdominal wall. The surgeon therefore makes an incision through the stretched skin, retrieves the navel (umbilicus), and sutures it into position.

While a sagging abdomen can be distressing in a male, so can enlarged breasts, particularly in a sensitive youngster. It is normal for a minor amount of breast enlargement to occur in the adolescent at puberty, but the excess usually disappears before the age of twenty-one. This relatively common occurrence of breast tissue in adolescent males is called gynecomastia; if the condition continues and the breasts become enlarged and abnormal in appearance after this age, deep-seated emotional problems can result. A teenager may be self-conscious about having physical attributes expected in only the opposite sex. His friends will surely notice any enlarged breast condition and subject him to unnecessary embarrassment.

Generally, surgery on the breasts is not recommended for an adolescent breast enlargement because in time the condition usually resolves itself, usually within two years. But if the condition should remain beyond adolescence, plastic surgery might be seriously considered. So far, there is no other remedy. Endocrine therapy has been tried but has not proven to be successful. Surgery is the most direct and effective method of treatment.

If a man should suddenly develop gynecomastia after his adolescence, he should be concerned about the cause. The enlargement may occur because of either benign or malignant tumors of the adrenal glands or the testes. In such a case health rather than cosmetic reasons obviously should be the primary concern. All possible causes of the breast enlargement should be investigated before any surgery is contemplated.

Contouring, or reducing the size of an abnormally large male breast, is fairly uncomplicated, although it usually requires hospitalization of approximately two to three days, general anesthesia, and, of course, the performance of a skilled surgeon. The operation is performed through an incision around the inferior half of the nipple through which the surgeon is able to core out fat and breast tissue and reshape the breast. This technique allows the surgeon to reduce the excess fat and breast tissue without extensive scarring; the scar is in the border between the nipple and the skin, and when healed is small and inconspicuous.

CASE HISTORIES

Steven, a nineteen-year-old college student, came to my office with his father. When I first met him, I wasn't sure why he had come; he was five feet eight inches tall and weighed about 180 pounds. As far as I could tell, he looked fine.

I discovered that Steven had once weighed 270 pounds, and that with the help of his family physician he was able to lose ninety pounds in about a year and a half. While he looked fine with clothes on, he had excess skin hanging from his abdomen. Despite a rigorous exercise program in conjunction with the weight loss he was not able to prevent the problem that he now faced. While his muscles were firm the abdominal skin was loose and bothersome to him. Steven was disturbed about his appearance—particularly embarrassed about being seen in the college locker room or in bathing trunks at the beach.

The first operation was performed on Steven's abdomen. All the excess skin and fat below his navel was removed. He has a scar from one side of his hipbone to the other, but his overall appearance is much improved, and the scar is hidden even when he is wearing bathing trunks. Steven realized that his weight loss was only the first step toward an improved appearance. The final step in his case was the cosmetic surgery that eliminated the unattractive aftereffects that massive weight loss often brings.

Ron is a twenty-one-year-old student who had an unusual but benign brain tumor as a youngster. The condition was successfully treated with cobalt radiation. The treatment, however, destroyed some of his body's normal endocrine mechanisms. In spite of a long-term hormonal replacement program, Ron had developed abnormally large breasts.

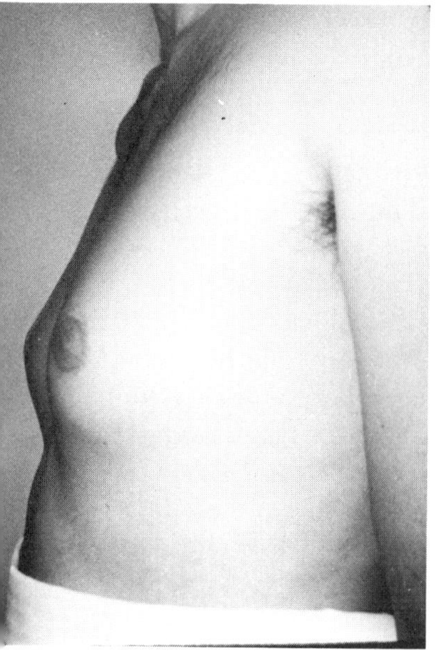

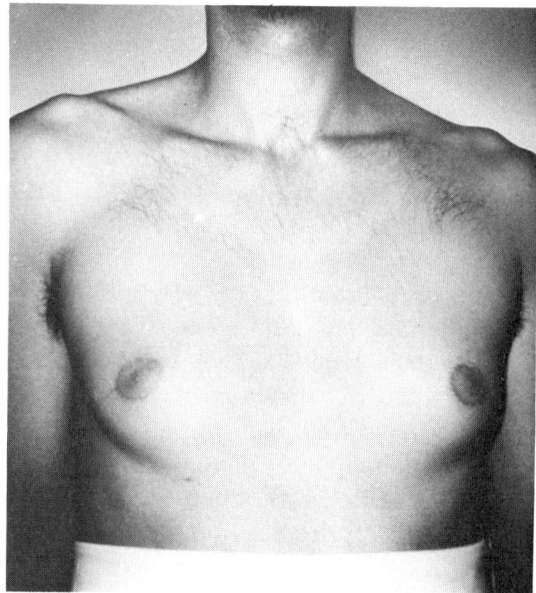

BEFORE

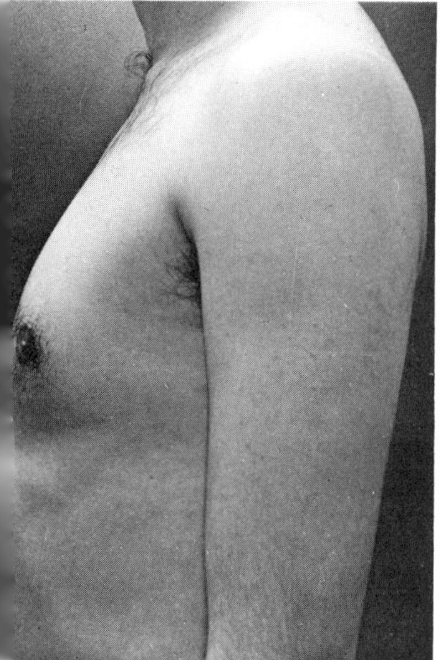

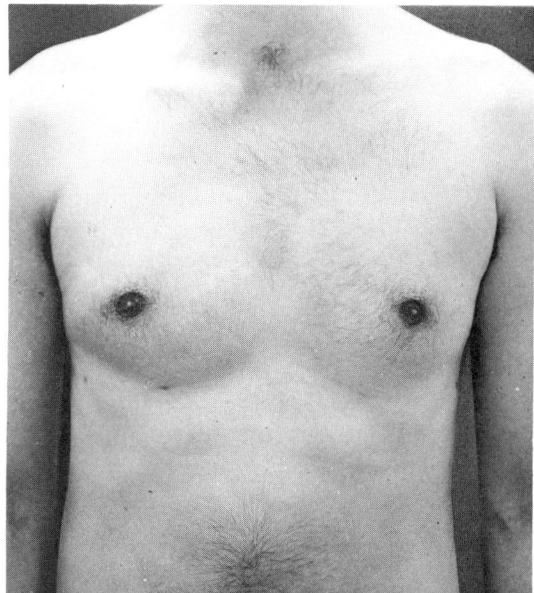

AFTER

Body Reduction (Gynecomastia)—Before and After

When Ron came to my office to discuss the problem, I told him I would have to confer with his endocrinologist. The endocrinologist approved of the operation, for in his opinion, this case of enlarged breasts would not resolve itself without surgical treatment. Through an incision around the inferior portion of the nipple, I was able to remove the excess fat and breast tissue. The skin then contracted to fit the new contour.

What constitutes "too much" fat in the breast area is often a subjective matter. One young man came to the office with a relatively minor amount of excess breast tissue. But someone he knew had made some uncomplimentary comments to him about his looking like a girl, which greatly upset him. Although the fat tissue was relatively minor, to this patient it was not, so I removed it. He is now content. Other men with seemingly large breasts couldn't care less, and often breast size is a relative matter of esthetics and concern.

There are also more unusual cases involving the restructuring of the breast. Dan, a twenty-seven-year-old economist, was born with a partially absent pectoral muscle under his existing left breast. As a result there was not only a depression in that area, but an abnormal fullness in his right breast—gynecomastia. An operation was performed on his enlarged breast to take away the fatty tissue. To build up the breast with the undeveloped muscle, an incision was made in the axilla, under the armpit area, and a custom-made Silastic implant, having previously been contoured to remedy the problem, was slipped under the minimally existent muscle fibers. The defect was thereby corrected and now Dan has relative symmetry of his two breasts.

SELF-EVALUATION

Only you can tell whether or not a body contouring procedure is for you, and whether it is a practical and reasonable answer to your problem. A full-length mirror is usually your best test, but there is another one you might also take. Get down on your hands and knees. Now, if there is redundant skin and fat hanging from your abdomen and you can hold or grab it between your fingertips and thumb, that excess can probably be removed surgically.

The question then arises as to whether surgery is medically recommended. If, for example, you have experienced a great weight loss, your plastic surgeon will want clearance from your physician before operating. Such weight loss might be accompanied by a variety of temporary changes in your cardiovascular system that could rule out surgery at the present time. It must be stressed that this surgery is usually for cases involving a great amount of weight loss.

Do not assume that abdominal lipectomy is meant to take off pounds if you are overweight. Most surgeons will not remove fat from men who have not first lost weight, for even if they did operate the results would be poor.

First, then, you must deal with the loss of weight through a sensible diet, preferably under a physician's care, before considering the surgical procedure. If after that you still have significant flab and excess skin, then something might be done to remove the effects surgically.

Whether you are a candidate for breast reduction depends on your own attitude. Most men feel that looking the least bit feminine is a stigma they cannot and will not accept. Some, however, are less sensitive about this condition.

THE PROCEDURES

Breast Reduction

In breast reduction, the "Webster incision," a half-moon made around the bottom part of the nipple, allows the surgeon to remove the excess fat and breast tissue. The surgeon can then dissect and remove as much breast tissue and fat as he needs to correct the problem. The bigger the breast, however, the more difficult it is for the stretched skin to shrink down normally afterwards. Usually excess skin will slowly shrink back in shape conforming to the new breast size. If there is still excess skin and a pendulous breast as a result of failure to conform to the new breast size, a secondary operation may have to be performed; in 90 percent of the cases, however, the skin will reconform by itself. The peri-areolar (half-moon) incision prevents noticeable incision scars. However, if redundant pendulous skin has to be removed the scars are longer and more noticeable—the price that sometimes must be paid.

When a breast is to be built up, such as in the case of the underde-

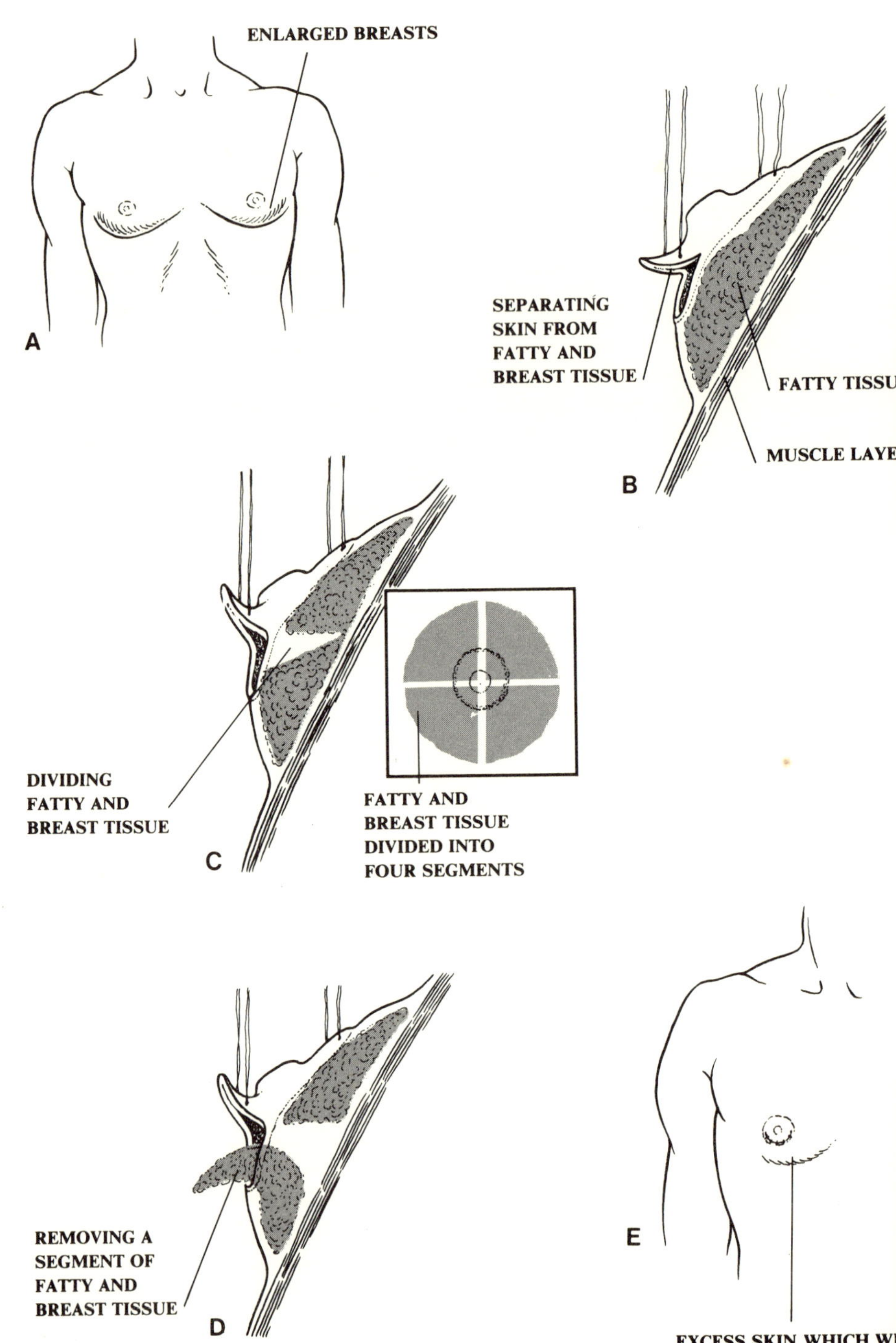
ENLARGED BREASTS
A
SEPARATING
SKIN FROM
FATTY AND
BREAST TISSUE
FATTY TISSU
MUSCLE LAYE
B
DIVIDING
FATTY AND
BREAST TISSUE
C
FATTY AND
BREAST TISSUE
DIVIDED INTO
FOUR SEGMENTS
REMOVING A
SEGMENT OF
FATTY AND
BREAST TISSUE
D
E
EXCESS SKIN WHICH W
CONFORM TO MUSCLE CONTO

veloped pectoral muscle, a Silastic implant can be used. This is custom made for each case. Using a special slow-curing plaster, the contour defect to be corrected is simulated and restructured. Plaster is then added to the area until the chest hollow is filled and the desired contour obtained. The edges are then feathered and smoothed and the plaster allowed to harden. This model is then sent to the surgical prosthesis company, which returns a Silastic version that can be of varying degrees of softness, depending on the specified areas and needs of the case. The implant is put into place, either through the nipple or the axilla (armpit).

Body Reduction

The entire procedure of an abdominal lipectomy takes about two hours. In preparation for abdominal lipectomy, the patient is shaved in the pubic area. The surgeon, with special skin-marking pen, then outlines the incision line on the abdomen and estimates the extent of skin removal. This is usually done while the patient is still standing, to get an accurate estimation of how much skin is to be removed, and to assure a straight incision line.

The patient is now placed under general anesthesia on the operating table. An incision is then made where the pen marks indicate—at the level of the pubic hairline and extending to the left and right sides of the lower abdomen to a point where the hipbones are prominent. The surgeon now separates and lifts the excess skin from the underlying muscle, excises the skin, and closes the wound. Reinforcement and correction of abdominal muscular weakness can also be corrected after the skin has been elevated.

In cutting away skin and closing the wound, the surgeon has to be

Opposite page: Body Reduction (Gynecomastia)

A. The female-appearing breast in a young male patient.
B. Profile view shows how the skin is separated from the underlying fatty and breast tissue.
C. The fatty tissue is usually removed in segments.
D. The fatty tissue being removed.
E. The final result. Notice that the only scar is around the inferior half of the nipple.

skillful in not cutting too much, or, for that matter, too little. If the skin is pulled too tight, complications can easily be caused by too much tension at the incision line. If the skin is too loose, the cosmetic improvement is not as great as it could have been.

AFTER SURGERY

Abdominal lipectomy requires about five to seven days' hospitalization. A drain, or catheter, is usually placed beneath the skin to collect any blood or other tissue fluids that might accumulate in the operative site. While the patient is convalescing in the hospital, the bed is jackknifed to between a 30- and 60-degree angle, so that tension is taken off the operative site, thus allowing healing to take place more easily. Bathroom privileges are usually granted within a day or two after surgery, at which time you can move around slowly. You will probably not be able to stand totally upright for several weeks, but within ten days to two weeks you should be able to return to work. Full participation in sports requires six weeks. Mild analgesics usually take care of any minor discomfort that might occur in the early postoperative periods.

After gynecomastia surgery the patient is usually kept in the hospital for a day or two. Discomfort is minimal, but there may be some ecchymosis (discoloration of the skin) as a result of the surgery. The swelling is minimal and what there is resolves itself in two or three weeks. The suction catheter that has been placed under the skin to collect any blood and tissue fluid is usually removed on the second postoperative day.

After surgery a light compression dressing is placed around the chest. Sutures are removed about a week to ten days after the operation. Because there probably will be some discomfort when the body

Opposite page: Body Reduction (Abdominal Lipectomy)

A. Profile view of redundant abdominal skin and fat.
B. The incision for the surgery is well below the bathing trunk line.
C. The skin is lifted away and the weakened abdominal muscles are tightened with sutures.
D. The excess skin and fat are removed.
E. The wound is closed and the navel is brought through an incision in the newly positioned skin.

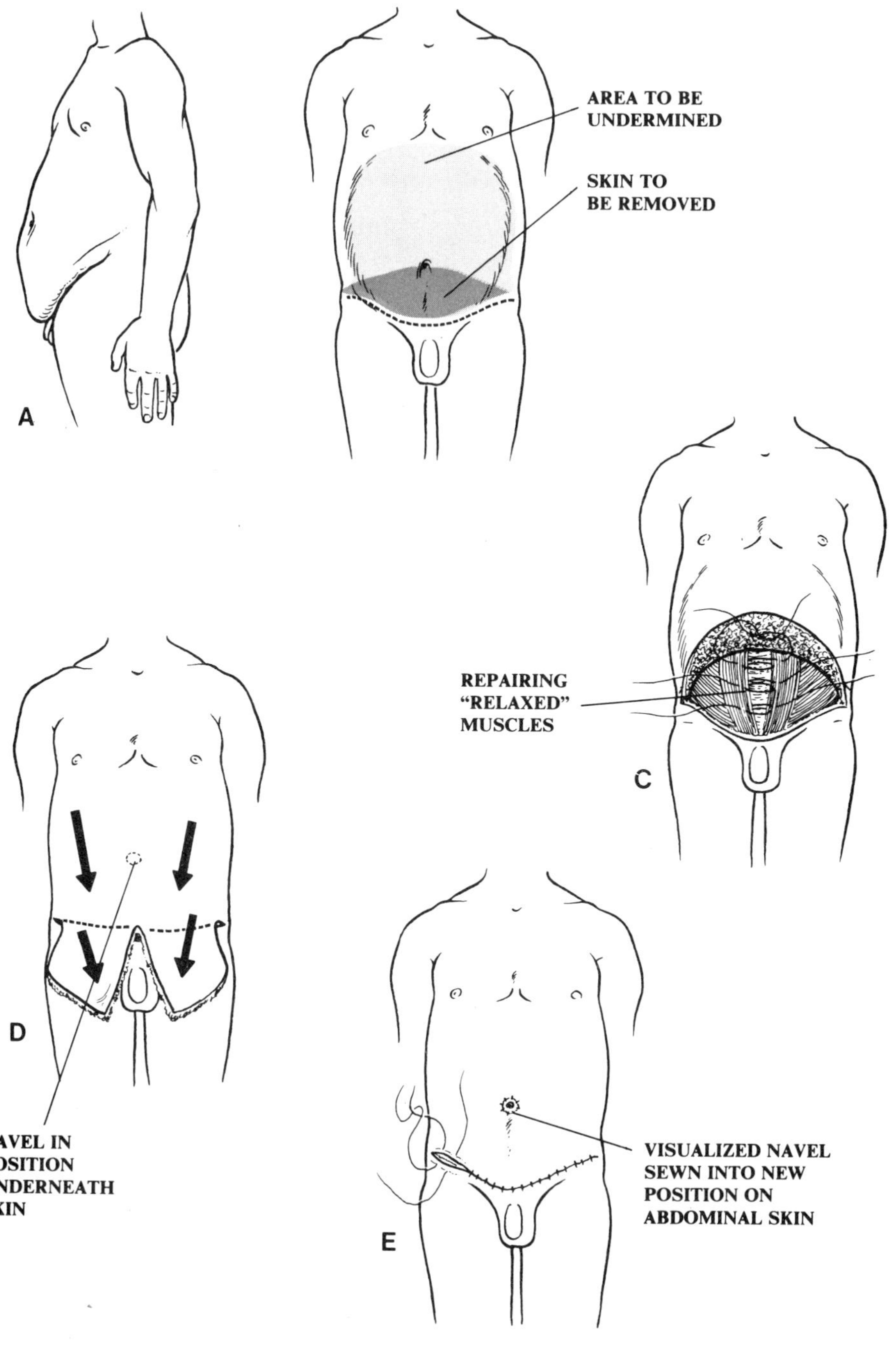
AREA TO BE
UNDERMINED
SKIN TO
BE REMOVED
A
REPAIRING
"RELAXED"
MUSCLES
C
D
AVEL IN
OSITION
NDERNEATH
KIN
VISUALIZED NAVEL
SEWN INTO NEW
POSITION ON
ABDOMINAL SKIN
E

is in motion, the patient generally waits a month after surgery before actively participating in sports.

WHAT CAN GO WRONG

Complications associated with abdominal lipectomy are rare. The most common postoperative problem is a widening of the scar. This happens because the skin is closed under moderate tension to secure the best cosmetic results; scar revision may have to be performed if the scar is excessively wide. Occasionally there is a small loss of skin, usually in the middle of the incision by the pubic area. Skin grafting is rarely necessary in such a case, because the problem will usually resolve itself and heal without incident.

The incision in surgery to correct gynecomastia is a small one. The operation is technically a cumbersome procedure; during the surgery bleeding can occur, and may be difficult to control through the small incision. When the breast tissue and fat are removed, there exists a potential space into which blood and tissue fluid could collect. A drainage catheter connected to a suction device can collapse the skin against the deeper tissue and thereby decrease the risk of hematoma—blood collection beneath the skin flaps. But despite the use of drainage tubes, blood can occasionally accumulate and an aspiration of the blood and any fluid may be necessary. This should not appreciably affect the outcome of the operation.

There might be a loss of sensation in the breast area after the operation, but this is a temporary condition. There may also be some moderate to severe bruising, but this too will resolve itself in a brief period of time.

Your surgeon will be careful not to remove all the breast and fat tissue, leaving behind enough to maintain a normal shape to the breast area. We specifically leave some tissue beneath the nipple so there will not be an unnatural looking depression beneath this area.

WHAT YOU CAN EXPECT

While you can expect an abdominal lipectomy to remove redundant skin and fat, it is not always possible to get rid of all the stretch marks. These usually result from the skin having been stretched for long periods of time. It is obvious that all of the abdominal skin cannot be removed by the surgery. The scar from the surgery will also be permanent. Most men, however, are quite pleased to have a more satisfying abdominal contour once the redundant skin and fat have been removed. The scar, which is well hidden, is a small price to pay.

Some men may wonder whether there will be a further problem if they once again gain weight after a skin-tightening operation. While I would hope that they would not gain excessively, there would be no major problems resulting from the surgical procedure, although the cosmetic effect would be lost. The skin can again stretch out. For instance, we do perform the operation on women who have stretched abdomens after pregnancy, even when they intend to become pregnant again.

TWELVE

Dermabrasion and Skin Planing

Dermabrasion, or skin planing, is a procedure utilizing a motor-driven rotating sander or disc. It enables the plastic surgeon to smooth down irregularities and contour defects of the skin that may have occurred as a result of the end stages of chicken pox, scars, and facial pits from acne, as well as accident scars.

The outer (epidermal) layer of skin is affected. It is removed during the process, while the upper part of the next (dermal) layer of the skin is only partially removed. This allows enough of the accessory skin structures, such as the sweat glands and minute hair follicles located in the deeper dermal layer, to remain and resurface the abraded areas. The skin surface is regenerated with little or minimal scarring.

From the original use of manually applied abrasive paper to the more sophisticated motor-driven instruments, the technique of dermabrasion has remained essentially the same over the last twenty or thirty years. Because the facial area has the greatest number of sweat glands and hair follicles, and because these elements reconstitute the skin surface after an abrasive process, the face—rather than the neck, back, or any other part of the body—is the most favorable area for successful dermabrasion.

The procedure involves planing the adjacent skin area so that the depth of any craters, pit marks, or scars becomes less apparent. The shallower the remaining scars and pits, the less noticeable they will appear when seen either outdoors or under harsher indoor lighting.

Dermabrasion is usually performed on scars, either surgical or traumatic in nature. The overall attempt or desired result is a leveling of the scar to the level of the surrounding skin so that they blend together making the scar less noticeable. Scars, or pit marks, as a result of chicken pox or end-stage acne can also be treated. Many of these cases, because of moderately deep scarring and pitting, may require a second or third abrasion. Unfortunately, situations that require second or third abrasions are the more severe ones. In such instances the third abrasion, although helpful, gives only minimal improvement compared to the first or second abrasion.

Dermabrasion has further use in the removal of tattoos. There are two types of tattoos. One is that done by either a professional or amateur. The amateur tattoo usually does not have the colored pigment imbedded in the deeper layers of the skin and will generally resolve itself fairly well; a superficial abrasion will expose the deeper particles and allow for their partial removal. The more professionally done tattoo, because of the skin depth to which the pigment has been placed, is not as readily treated by dermabrasion; frequently it may be removed by excision of the offending tattoo and use of a split-thickness skin graft or by serial (a series) excision of the tattoo if it isn't too large.

A second type of tattoo scar is called an "accidental tattoo." It is formed when an individual sustains an injury (frequently in an automobile accident) and is thrown to the side of the road or to the sidewalk, abrading the skin. Foreign matter—dirt, various particles, especially road tar—may be imbedded in the skin. Unless adequately removed at the time of the accident, when the skin resurfaces in the abraded area the particles may be trapped beneath this new layer of skin. The disfigurement can be improved by dermabrasion. Reabrading the area will reexpose the particles, allowing their removal.

Dermabrasion is also used in the treatment of fine wrinkles in and around the upper and lower lip. These lines and wrinkles are softened by leveling the surrounding skin or by a technique I prefer—which will be discussed later in this chapter—called chemical peeling.

The Acute Acne Conditon

For patients with acute acne, dermabrasion is not the answer. I will usually refer such persons to a dermatologist who can treat them until the condition is under control; only then can they be candidates for surgery. Frequently, patients with acute acne consult with me anyway, in the anticipation that dermabrasion will cure or at least arrest the acne condition. We reserve abrasion for cases in which the acne has been brought under control and only end-stage pitting mars the face.

PROCEDURE

Dermabrasion can be performed either on an outpatient basis or during a short stay in the hospital. If the latter, a general anesthetic can be administered; this avoids the direct injection of a numbing solution or the application of a commercial freezing solution to numb the facial skin.

I usually prefer the general anesthetic, particularly for full face abrasion. However, with adequate preoperative sedation, followed by an injection of novocaine or application of a chemical coolant, dermabrasion can also be performed comfortably under local anesthesia.

Regardless of what type of anesthesia is used, the technique—as mentioned above—involves the removal of the upper layer of skin, leaving the deeper tissues to regenerate and resurface the abraded area. Approximately five to seven days are required for a new skin layer to regenerate. Initially there is a serum or crust that develops over the abraded area, under which cellular activity increases in the resurfacing process.

Chemical Peeling

Chemical peeling, or chemosurgery, is a process involving the application of a caustic solution, such as phenol or a trichloracetic acid, to the skin. The result: the sloughing off or loss of the epidermal layer, with some of the superficial part of the skin's dermal layer. Upon healing, many of the fine lines or wrinkles of the face can be removed. The technique is also beneficial in removing some of the brown-pigmented aging spots frequently seen on the face. However, I have seen cases where caustic agents were applied by nonmedical personnel, with destructive results and terrible scarring.

While trichloracetic acid has been used in this country, the more common technique is the use of phenol, a chemical caustic agent

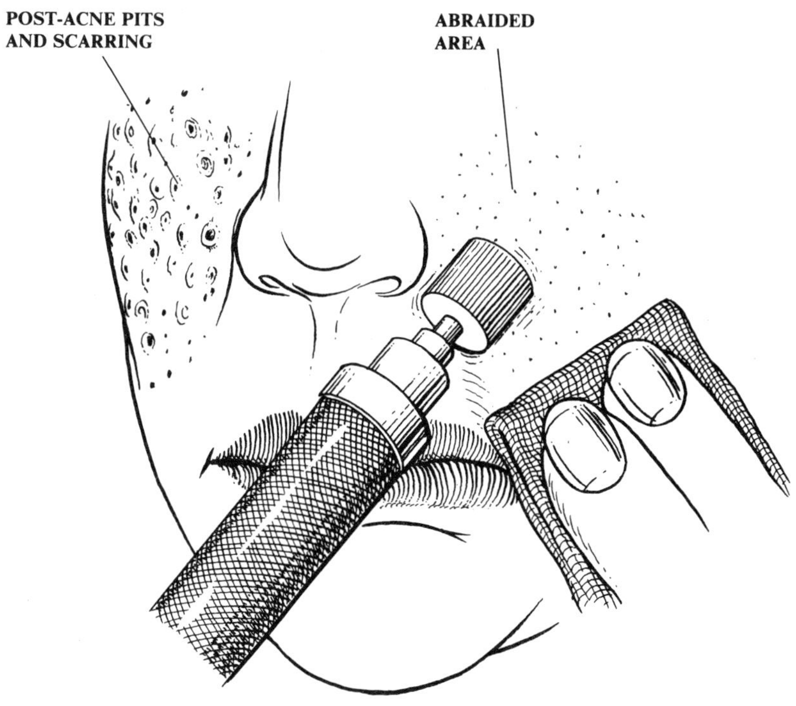

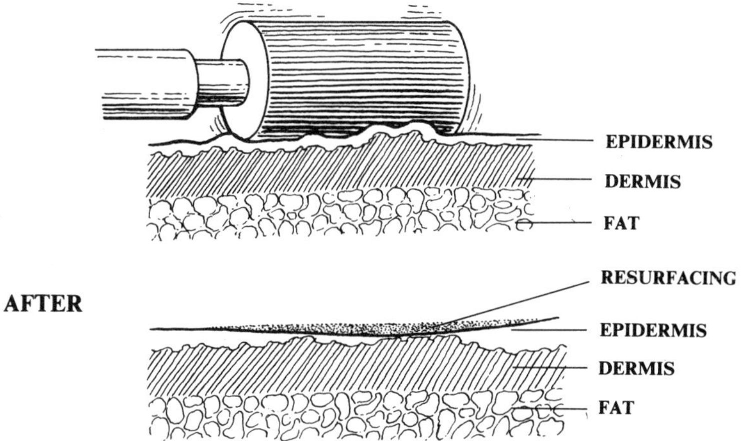

Dermabrasion

that works in a process similar to mechanical abrasion. The application of phenol will result in the removal of the epidermal (upper) layer, and part of the dermal, or next, layer of the skin by a coagulation process. The resurfacing of this peeled area, with a new layer of skin, occurs in five to seven days. As in the dermabrasion process, the accessory skin structures (hair follicles and sweat glands) located in the deeper layers of the skin are responsible for the resurfacing of the new skin layer.

During chemical peeling one of the more interesting changes occurs in the deeper layers of the skin, and as a result of the process there appears to be a thickening of these deeper layers. Microscopic examination of the skin where the process has been performed shows a reorientation of the collagen fibers, and possibly an increase in the stability, quantity, and quality of the elastic fibers in the new skin layer. These factors, combined with the newly resurfaced skin, are responsible for a more youthful appearance.

In addition to the changes in the collagen and elastic fibers of the skin, there are also changes in the pigmentary granules in the skin's basal layer. These are responsible for the occasional bleaching or pigmentary changes of the skin following chemical peeling. Permanent bleaching or discoloration of the skin is not the desired result; this occurs more frequently with darker-skinned individuals, and for that reason not every patient is a candidate for this procedure.

Chemical peeling is usually performed as an adjunct to face-lift and/or eye surgery in an attempt to get rid of many of the fine lines around the eyes and mouth—specifically, though, the upper and lower lips.

Patients who have multiple fine lines around the eyes and mouth will benefit from the peeling simply because face- and eye-lift surgery isn't designed to remove such fine facial wrinkles. The entire face can be peeled, or selected areas such as the upper and lower lips and the eyelids may be chosen for treatment. Each case is individual and your surgeon will discuss your particular needs with you.

The surgical procedure can be performed on an in-patient or out-patient basis. General anesthesia is usually not necessary. The area to be peeled is prepped with a pHisoHex soap solution, after which acetone is applied. This helps dissolve the natural fats and oils of the skin to allow for good penetration of the phenol solution. Phenol is applied with a Q-Tip and distributed symmetrically over the entire face, or the area to be treated. There may be an initial burning sensation as it is applied to the skin, but this lasts only a few minutes and then disappears. After phenol has been applied, I use a waterproof tape in small strips, measuring from one half to three inches in length. This forms a facial mask over the area that has been treated with the chemical; it stays on for approximately two days and then is removed. At this time there may be some oozing, and a general hue of redness can appear on the face as a result of the phenol's action. For this, I usually dust a powder of thymol iodine over the entire area. Applied daily, for approximately one to two days, it will help form a coagulum, or crust, in the operated area. Approximately two or three days after surgery, I begin applications of cold cream. (By the way, commercial Crisco is quite acceptable.) In approximately a week to ten days the incrustation is gone.

Over the next three- to four-week period the surface has healed to such a degree that the patient is able to apply makeup to camouflage the redness, which will persist for some time. Gentle cleansing of the face with a mild soap is possible within a week to ten days. Of course, direct exposure to the sun should be avoided for at least three to six months, and after that time caution should be taken to avoid sunburn. I usually advise the use of a sun-blocking agent.

Minor problems that develop are similar for both dermabrasion and chemical peeling. There is the appearance of milia, or whiteheads, which usually respond to cleansing with a mild abrasive soap. Other problems that may occur (other than the rare occurrence of a thickened scar) are demarcations from peeled to unpeeled areas. Peeling ends at the jawline and is not carried out on the neck. (Chemical peeling of the neck can increase the possibility of thickened scars and so the peeling process is not continued in this sensitive area.) Therefore, there will be an area of contrast. There may also be some demarcation between face and the surrounding upper and lower lip areas, if these are treated without peeling the entire face. A peri-oral peel merely treats the lips; without treating the rest of the face, a faintly whitish discolored area may appear around the upper and lower lips. Because this discoloration may be prominent, many surgeons will chemically treat only the forehead, nose, and upper lip as one unit, leaving the lower lip unabraded or un-

untreated with a chemical. If the entire face is done, there is a possibility that pigmentary changes might occur.

AFTER SURGERY

Full facial dermabrasion takes approximately one hour. After the process of abrasion is performed, any deeper pits that the surgeon feels will not respond to treatment can be excised at that time. These pits, when treated by excision, are transformed into small linear scars that are less unsightly, for a straight-leveled scar will always be less noticeable than a recessed crater.

I usually apply a non-sticking gauze dressing to the abraded area. This is later soaked off, generally within seventy-two to ninety-six hours, by application of a saline solution. In some cases, however, the gauze layer may remain for approximately five to seven days before a spontaneous separation occurs. In either case the abraded area is usually healed by then. During this period the new skin cover is beginning to re-form by the natural action of the small cellular units (sweat glands and hair follicles) that have been allowed to remain within the deeper layers of the skin. The new epidermal cells that form will resurface the skin; certainly in ten to fourteen days all of the superficial crusting is completely off and, on the facial area, although healed, a reddish color appears. This redness slowly resolves itself within a few weeks. I frequently recommend the application of a steroid cream, which will help decrease the redness. At this point a light makeup lotion or thin covering of powder can be applied. Most patients return to work within two weeks—with considerable visible improvement.

In the initial postoperative period of approximately two to three weeks, there will be moderate swelling. This gives the impression of smooth skin and indicates the possibility of a good result. Unfortunately, as the swelling decreases, some of the initial visible good results begin to disappear—much to the dismay of the patient as well as the physician. I explain this to the patient beforehand, so that his expectations will be realistic and he will suffer no great disappointment if the results are less than perfect.

Pigmentary changes are a problem, particularly in darker-complected Caucasians and black males. Skin color is due in large part to the number and concentration of the melanin, or pigment-containing, granules in the basal, or deeper, layers of the skin. The darker our skin complexion, the more melanin granules are present. In the first few weeks after the abrasion, there is little change in the pigment of the skin, but with the passage of time, repigmentation usually increases as a result of the stimulus of surgery. This accounts for the initial darkening of the skin in the abraded area, followed by a lightening of the area as the hyperpigmentation fades. The increase may not be uniform and could result in some hyperpigmented areas in contrast to the surrounding skin color. Repigmentation can also be accentuated by exposure to the sun; therefore, I advise that a sun-screen lotion rather than a suntan lotion be applied to the face for several months after the surgery, particularly when direct exposure to the sun is a possibility. As time goes on, the intensity of color will fade, but in some areas spotty pigmentary changes may remain. Increases and/or decreases in pigment are less noticeable in fair-skinned patients, but more so in those with darker skins. And so for those patients in whom we can anticipate a significant color difference, we take great pains to fully explain such a possibility. In some individuals—such as blacks—dermabrasion is often not advised because of the predictability of significant color differences that result from the procedure.

WHAT YOU CAN EXPECT

It is now several weeks since the surgical procedure and the healing is nearly complete. The swelling is resolving, and while the redness is still there, it is fading with time. At this stage the improvement from the surgery is quite visible; nevertheless, it has a tendency to be slightly less than what the patient may have expected. Once the initial swelling has resolved itself, some of the moderately deep pits that could not be removed by dermabrasion resurface and become visible again, though less noticeable than before.

At this point it is important to recognize that a second and third abrasion may be necessary. If this is a possibility, it will have been discussed with you beforehand. I believe it very important to inform prospective candidates at the initial consultation that more than one procedure may be needed for maximum improvement. Obviously, more procedures are necessary in severe post-acne scarring; here again, the results depend on the initial condition. It is my belief that after two or three abrasions the maximum results will have probably been obtained. Dermabrasion can accomplish just so much. It has been designed to improve superficial and some deeper acne scars, but in no way can it give totally smooth skin. Patients with deeper scarring will require multiple abrasions. They will get improvement, but certainly less favorable end results than those cases with only superficial pitting.

Chemical Peeling

As mentioned above, the patient who has a chemical peel should avoid direct sunlight for a period of three to six months. Failure to do this may increase the potential for irregular discolored areas and patches. If the phenol solution has been applied evenly over the entire face, it should result in very minimal color differences over the treated area. However, should irregular, patchy discolored areas occur they will usually resolve themselves within several months. Further, any unresolved areas of discoloration may respond to a secondary peeling. Occasionally, as with all these procedures, there may be some permanent discoloration. In these cases it may be covered with makeup. Finally, to repeat an earlier caution, this procedure is not recommended for those individuals subject to pigmentary changes—dark-skinned Caucasians and, of course, blacks.

THIRTEEN

Penile and Testicular Implants

PLASTIC SURGERY is performed in the male genital area to resolve problems related to birth defects and other physical abnormalities. These defects often involve the urethra—the tube that extends from the bladder through the penis to convey urine. Injury to the genitalia from traumatic causes, such as the devastation of war and injury through accidents, can also be treated surgically.

Surgery has also been employed successfully to help an impotent male achieve an erection. Finally, plastic surgery is utilized for men, not in the usual sense of re-creating part of the anatomy, but rather eliminating it—through the mechanics of transsexual operations.

BIRTH DEFECTS

Sexual characteristics of the human embryo are not visible until the eighth or tenth week of development. Before this stage there is a mass of "sexless" tissue in that area where the genitalia will develop. Genitalia are evident in the embryo after the second month by the development of the Mullerian (female) or Wolffian (male) ducts. In the male embryo the Mullerian duct atrophies and disappears, while the Wolffian duct continues to grow and forms part of the ejaculatory system. The opposite happens to the female embryo as its sex characteristics develop. Here, the Wolffian duct atrophies while the Mullerian duct continues to develop into the uterus, oviduct, and vagina.

In some cases, the male embryo may develop in an abnormal manner that will cause problems with the infant's genitalia; one such condition is called epispadias, in which the urethra opens up at the upper surface of the penis. Another condition, called hypospadias, occurs when the urethra opens up on the undersurface of the

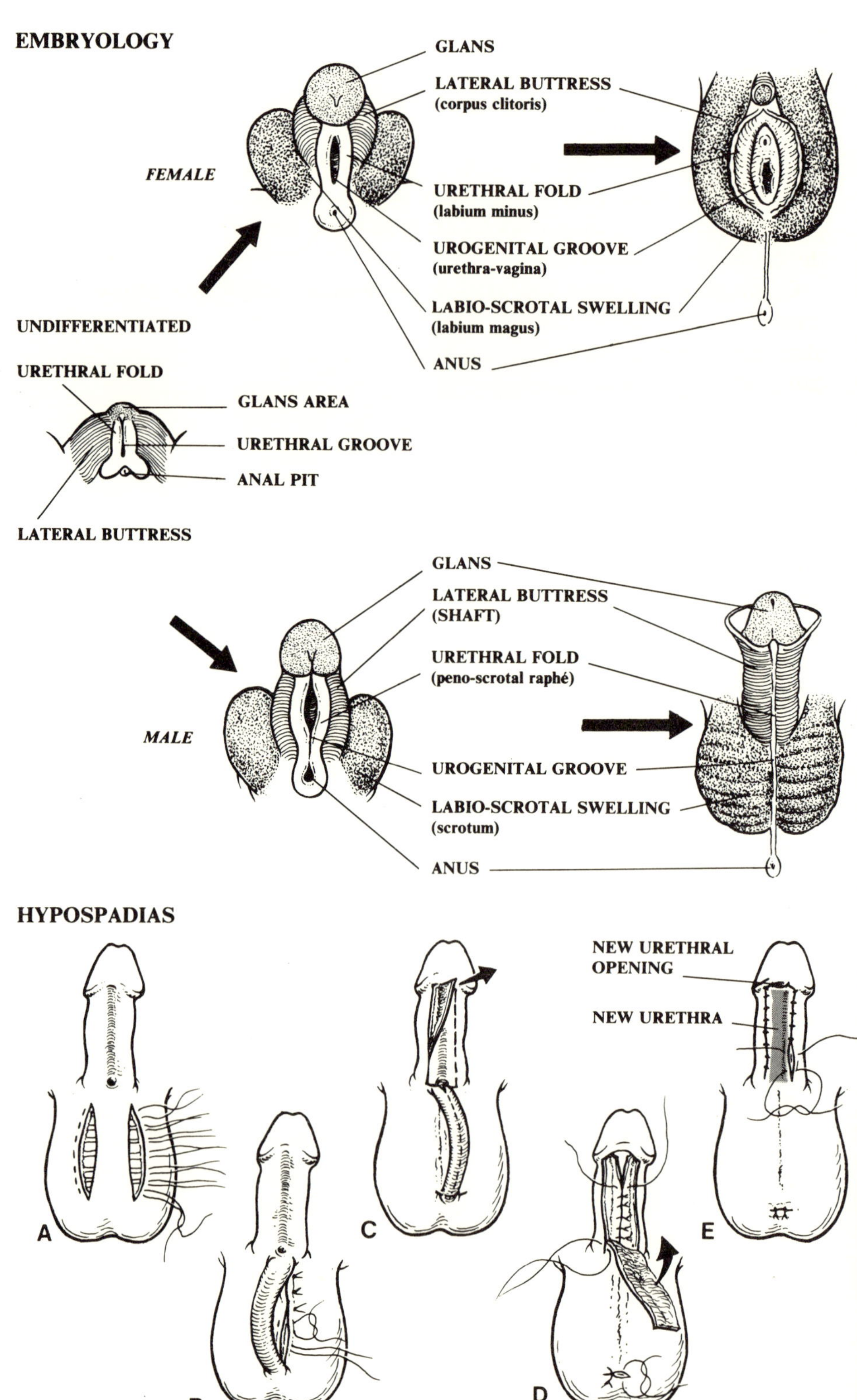

EMBRYOLOGY
GLANS
LATERAL BUTTRESS
(corpus clitoris)
FEMALE
URETHRAL FOLD
(labium minus)
UROGENITAL GROOVE
(urethra-vagina)
LABIO-SCROTAL SWELLING
(labium magus)
ANUS
UNDIFFERENTIATED
URETHRAL FOLD
GLANS AREA
URETHRAL GROOVE
ANAL PIT
LATERAL BUTTRESS
GLANS
LATERAL BUTTRESS
(SHAFT)
URETHRAL FOLD
(peno-scrotal raphé)
MALE
UROGENITAL GROOVE
LABIO-SCROTAL SWELLING
(scrotum)
ANUS
HYPOSPADIAS
NEW URETHRAL
OPENING
NEW URETHRA
A
B
C
D
E

penis, almost in the scrotal area. A still rarer situation is one in which the bladder actually is situated outside the abdominal wall.

All of these conditions are correctible to a variable degree by surgery. Procedures to lengthen or redirect the urethra are considered complex, but when performed under the direction of a competent plastic surgeon or urologist specializing in these areas of correction, the result can be gratifying.

Operations to correct the urethra are usually performed before school age. The penis generally is large enough by the age of two; also, at this age psychological problems have not yet developed because of the penile abnormality.

ABNORMALITIES THAT DEVELOP LATER

Not all problems related to the penis are congenital. It may happen that the testes will not descend and remain in the abdomen. If that abnormality is not corrected early enough, atrophy may occur and an individual might end up with only one testicle, or at least one, smaller than normal, which may not function.

A plastic surgeon can simulate a testicle with a Silastic implant when the testicle has not developed normally or if it has been lost as a result of injury, such as that caused by an automobile accident, gunshot wound, or war-related incident. These implants are made in sizes that are suitable for both youngsters and adults. The operation, however, has only a cosmetic effect; the implant cannot function as a testicle.

Opposite page: Penile and Testicular Implants

Embryology: *The embryology of the male and female reproductive system starts out similar to each other, but each goes on to develop into the unique sexual apparatus of the male or female.*

Hypospadias:

A. The urethra doesn't reach to the tip of the penis, a congenital abnormality.

B. A tube of skin is created from the scrotum and is used to lengthen the congenitally shortened urethra, finally allowing it to function normally.

C–D. A tube of skin re-creates the shortened urethra.

E. The urine stream can now reach the tip of the penis.

If the genital area itself is mutilated as a result of an accident, trauma, or injury, a number of procedures can be used to reconstruct the area.

Another condition that can occur in the adult male is called Peronies's disease, since it was first described in 1819 by François de la Peronies, the physician to Louis XIV. The disease also has other names, including plastic induration, fibrous plaque, or fibrous sclerosis of the penis. With this condition, plaque is formed on the dorsum, or top, of the penis; it can vary in length and thickness or it can exist as a core or nodule. Because of this thickening of the skin, there is an unusual curvature when the penis is erect, thereby causing extreme discomfort. At the same time, the existence of the plaque is painless when the penis is in the flaccid state.

While Peronies's disease is most frequently seen in men between forty and sixty, it also occurs in both older and younger patients. Treatment varies, as do the results. Some patients receive systematic treatments of potassium para-amino-benzoate; others have been treated with steroids. Surgical removal of the plaque is successful in some cases without any type of reconstruction being necessary, while in other cases more extensive surgery is required. Surgery frees up the contracture of the tissue and the curvature of the erect penis is thus corrected. A skin graft may also be placed on the site to help prevent the problem from recurring.

IMPOTENCE

The mechanism of coitus, which begins with libido and erection and then terminates with ejaculation and orgasm, is a most complex system. It combines a low spinal reflex and a high cortical reflex as well as an important psychic element. However complicated this mechanism can be, one item is essential to the sexual act: the ability of the man to insert his penis inside the vagina of his female partner. Failure to do so will create a psychological climate of tension and anxiety and the onset of impotency, while the ability to introduce the penis can give the man the self-confidence that will encourage normal completion of the act.

There are two types of impotence: psychological and organic. Psychological impotence is the most common circumstance, occurring in more than 95 percent of such cases. It is often difficult to find the underlying conflict that causes it, but it can be cured in many instances. Organic impotence may also be corrected if the cause is found and treated. This type of impotence can be caused by diseases of the nervous system as well as by obesity, diabetes, and post-surgical defects that cause fistulas of the urinary tract. There have been estimates that over one million men in the United States are impotent from diabetes alone.

Impotence can also be the result of surgery performed on patients who have cancer of the prostate, bladder, colon, or rectum; if the nerves have been damaged or cut as a necessary part of the ablative surgery, a normal erection would not be possible.

Vascular problems can also cause impotence. A situation called Reisch syndrome occurs when there is a blockage of the aorta—the major blood vessel from the heart that eventually splits into left and right vessels supplying the lower extremities. When the blood that is supposed to go to the groin area is blocked because of the arteriosclerotic process that occurs as we get older, impotency can occur. Vascular problems, however, can often be corrected with a bypass operation, allowing return of sexual function in some instances.

A man with a vascular impairment may very well think that his impotency is purely psychological, when actually there are physical causes. It is therefore vital that he have a complete physical checkup when there is a sudden occurrence of impotency—particularly when the man is between forty and fifty years of age. In some cases there could be an invasive carcinoma in the area that impinges on the nerves necessary to bring on an erection. Impotency has also occurred in men who have suffered pelvic fractures, ruptured urethras, and other urological problems following fractures of the vertebral and pelvic area.

It is important to note that even though only 5 percent of impotency problems have medical roots—post-cancer operations, radical operations on the prostate, multiple sclerosis, neurological problems, and sometimes diabetes—you should not automatically assume you are in the 95-percent category. Get a medical checkup. A urologist is perhaps the specialist most familiar with medical problems associated with impotence.

Assuming that you don't have a treatable medical problem, and if your impotency has not been helped through psychological counseling, you then might consider treating your impotence through plastic surgery.

Treatment of Impotence

An accepted surgical technique for treating impotency is the insertion of a polyethylene rod in the penis. The rod is introduced beneath the skin on either side of what is termed the corpus cavernosum. It is placed deep enough so that there will be little possibility of extrusion and so pressure-sensitivity of the rod on the skin will not be a problem.

The effect of the rod is to imitate a natural erection that is normally caused by the filling of the corpus cavernosum with blood. The surgeon makes an incision along the base or root of the penis and passes the rod down the entire length into the tip. Not completely to the tip, though, because you don't want to have it extruding or pushing through. The implant is made of Silastic—the same Silastic made for chin, nose, and breast implants, just a harder version. It is not brittle, so it is not breakable. There is an inflatable version available, its advantage being, of course, that the penis would not have to be erect all the time. All the ramifications of this procedure will be discussed with you by your surgeon.

TRANSSEXUAL OPERATIONS

Sex-change operations have been reported to be on the increase at some major medical centers around the country. Changes are made to and from both sexes: male to female and female to male. (There are a certain number of males—probably between 1:50,000 and 1:100,000—who may be candidates for transsexual operations.) When a patient goes to the gender identity clinic of a medical center to have his sex changed, he doesn't just make an appointment with a surgeon. There is a period of intense psychological and social counseling. Surgery is just one part of the transformation. After all, it's a once-in-a-lifetime procedure. When it's done, there's no turning back.

Most gender identity clinics involved in transsexual surgery will

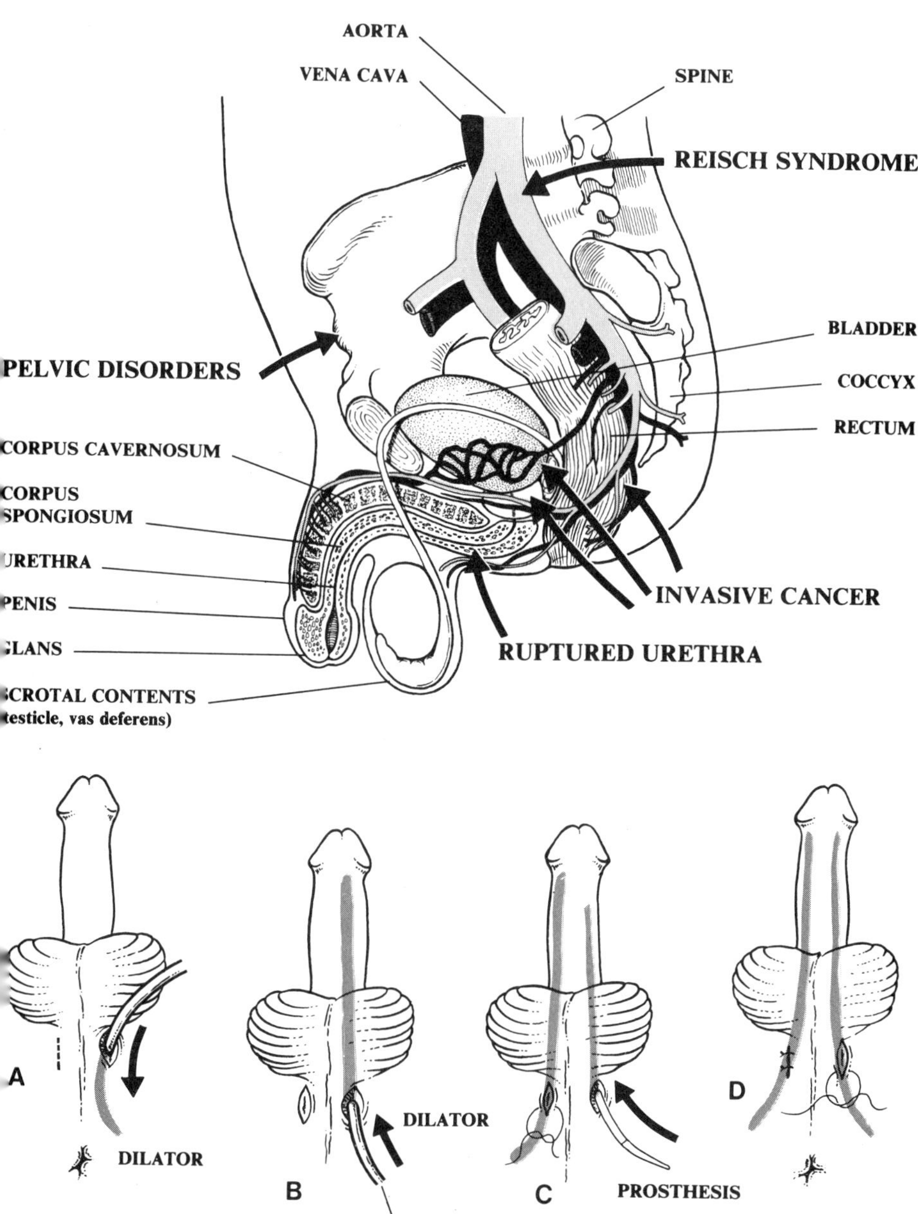

The Anatomy of the Male Genital System and Correction of Impotence

Above: *Some of the causes of impotence are pelvic disorders, Reisch syndrome, a ruptured urethra, and invasive cancer.*

Below: The penile implant

A. A dilator is inserted.

B. After the dilator has formed a tunnel, the Silastic rod is inserted.

C. A second Silastic rod is inserted.

D. The result, with two Silastic rods in place.

require that the patient live the life of the other sex for at least a year or more before the operation. Psychiatric treatment before the surgery is uniformly recommended. The doctor will work with the patient until he has explored all avenues of therapy and then, if the patient still persists, the operation—the removal of the penis and testicles and the construction of an artificial vagina—can be performed by a plastic surgeon and a urologist. The newly formed vagina will have some limited sensory capabilities because it is essentially reconstructed from the male genital organ.

The female transsexual who wishes to become a man requires multiple surgical procedures before the final transformation is accomplished. The penis has no sensate capacity. It is artificially constructed of Silastic material within a skin tube created from either the abdomen or thigh and cannot experience normal sensation. Its only function is as an organ to be inserted.

The work preparatory to this operation—the testing to make sure that the patient is ready for the surgery—is every bit as important a part of the procedure as the operation itself. It would be wise to consult with a specialist in this field before considering such surgery.

Because of the complex psychological and emotional factors involved, I feel these procedures should be performed in a university setting where all the involved medical and surgical disciplines are available.

FOURTEEN

Nonesthetic Surgery

NOT ALL plastic surgery is elective and purely cosmetic. Often the skills of a plastic surgeon are required in emergency situations, such as after an accident. Some birth defects also require the services of a plastic surgeon, as does reconstruction following removal of a variety of tumors, usually from around the area of the head and neck.

CASE HISTORIES

Accidents are particularly challenging to a plastic surgeon. There is not much time to analyze and study a case. I arrive at the hospital, look at the patient, get as much information as I can, and immediately start placing the pieces of the body together again.

I was called on a case one New Year's Eve to tend to an eighteen-year-old boy who was injured in an automobile accident. His nose was quite swollen and bloody when I first saw him, but on the whole he didn't look too bad. In the emergency room, though, I could see that the nose was held together by only clots of blood, and could be opened up the way you would open a book. I didn't realize the magnitude of the problem, though, until I started to lift away the blood clots. It then was obvious that the nose was partially amputated and being kept alive by only a narrow rim of tissue.

The entire operation took only forty-five minutes. At first it looked as if it would be a much lengthier procedure, but while complex and difficult, it went along quickly without complications. The boy was given a local anesthetic, the wound was irrigated, the broken bones were reset, and the skin was unfolded and placed in the proper position. The nose was stitched on the outside, and also from within the nostril.

Remarkably good results were evident from the very beginning. I saw David nine months later and, deciding that the scar was a little irregular, I sanded it. Today David has a very fine linear scar going from the top of his nose down to the nostril. Considering the extent of his injury—essentially his nose had been amputated—the scarring is minimal indeed.

Anyone who ignores cancerous growths for a long time is asking for trouble. Harold, a fifty-three-year-old salesman, came to my office after being referred to me by his family physician. Harold had a growth on his nose between the nostrils. He said that the growth had been there only a few weeks, but his wife volunteered that he had probably had it for at least six months.

My examination showed that the lesion was growing not only on the inside of the nostrils, but also on the outside and up the tip of the nose. While the area looked no bigger than a dime, the surgical procedure was going to be complicated. Assuming, as I did, that the growth was malignant, the lesion would have to be cut out along with some normal skin around it, to make sure that the malignancy was completely excised. The columella—the separation between the nostrils—would have to be taken off along with the entire tip of the nose.

While I assumed that the growth was a carcinoma, I wasn't going to cut off most of Harold's nose until I was absolutely sure. He was taken to the hospital where a biopsy was performed. The pathologist's report indicated basal cell carcinoma. Because the tumor was infiltrating deep, I had to go wide around the lesion to cut it out. I kept sending sections down to the pathology department until they finally said that they had normal skin, which meant that the tumor had been removed.

The tumor wasn't the type that spreads throughout the body, so Harold was "cured." But that was only part of the battle. There was a big hole where a nose used to be, and it had to be reconstructed. What I did was develop some bulk for the site by first taking some skin from the adjacent cheek area, elevating it, folding it, and turning it in to restore some semblance of a normal looking nose. Harold will be having several operations before the procedure is completed. The sad thing is that all of the operations wouldn't have been necessary if he had gone to a physician earlier. Less tissue would have had to be removed and the reconstruction would have been much less complicated.

A thirty-two-year-old physician in one of the hospitals with which I am affiliated also had a lesion on his nose. It was probably the result of radiation to which he was exposed when young. Throughout his life he had recurrent skin tumors in the nasal area, and as each was removed more of the nose was removed along with it.

When the doctor was referred to me, he needed additional surgery, but it couldn't be determined how much tissue had to be taken off. We took him to the operating room, administered a general anesthesia, and kept removing tissue until the pathologists assured me that all of the cancerous cells were removed.

By the time the operation was over more than half the skin and cartilage of his nose had been taken away. Nose reconstruction was started immediately, so that he wouldn't be left with a large defect in the middle of his nose. Reconstruction began by taking skin from the cheek fold, elevating it, and rotating it into position. The doctor-patient was discharged but came back in a couple of weeks to have this skin contoured and further shaped into a nose. It's been a year since I operated on him. There has been no recurrence of his disease, and his restructured nose looks normal.

CONDITIONS REQUIRING NONESTHETIC SURGERY; METHODS OF TREATMENT

Injuries to the Skin

In accidents where the skin is avulsed or torn away, leaving an open raw area, it's possible, if the area isn't very large, for the skin to resurface with a new layer, even though it may take a long time. As an alternative, a skin graft can be placed over the wound. The grafted skin probably will come from the buttocks or thighs.

When a patch of skin is taken away from the body, it will leave a discolored area. If it is taken from an area like the buttocks, this area is generally hidden from view, even if the person is wearing bathing trunks. So when the appearance of the face, arms, or legs can be improved, the tradeoff is a good one.

Instead of using a skin graft in such a situation, the surgeon may use a variety of techniques to rotate locally available tissue within the same area to cover the defect. Because skin grafts are cut off and moved from one part of the body to another, a new blood supply can be reestablished only with very thin skin, up to 22/1000 inch. Skin grafts rarely approach the thickness of the segments they are replacing. In the facial area, a depression in relation to the surrounding normal area will look cosmetically better if local tissue similar in thickness to that which has been removed is utilized. Therefore local flaps are used. These give excellent contour restoration.

The newest method of skin transfer is the microvascular technique, in which the surgeon takes skin as well as fat and even underlying muscle from an area, such as the groin, where specific blood vessels supply the skin and fat. An area about the size of a pancake, up to four inches in diameter, is outlined. The major feeding arteries and veins are dissected, and the pancake of tissue is cut, preserving the vessels that supply it. The whole area is picked up, cut free from the body, and taken up to the facial area where it is sutured into some major blood vessel in the face or neck area. The surgeon, aided by a microscope, takes fine suture material and sews the blood vessels together. It is an amazing feat; some of the blood vessels are only one to two millimeters in diameter.

Microvascular technology is being used increasingly to transplant large composites of tissue from one area to another in one stage. The older method required forming a tube of skin in the groin area, and ultimately attaching it onto the arm, and slowly waltzing it up to the face. The skin got its blood supply from each new area. The new one-step method, while trickier and more involved, could well be the surgery of the future.

Burns

Injuries from burns present special problems for the plastic surgeon. No matter how the injury is taken care of there will be a discoloration and thickening of the new skin in the burnt area. So far, there's nothing that can be done about that. Surgeons can only concentrate on the restoration of the skin's function and decrease the mortality from severe burns.

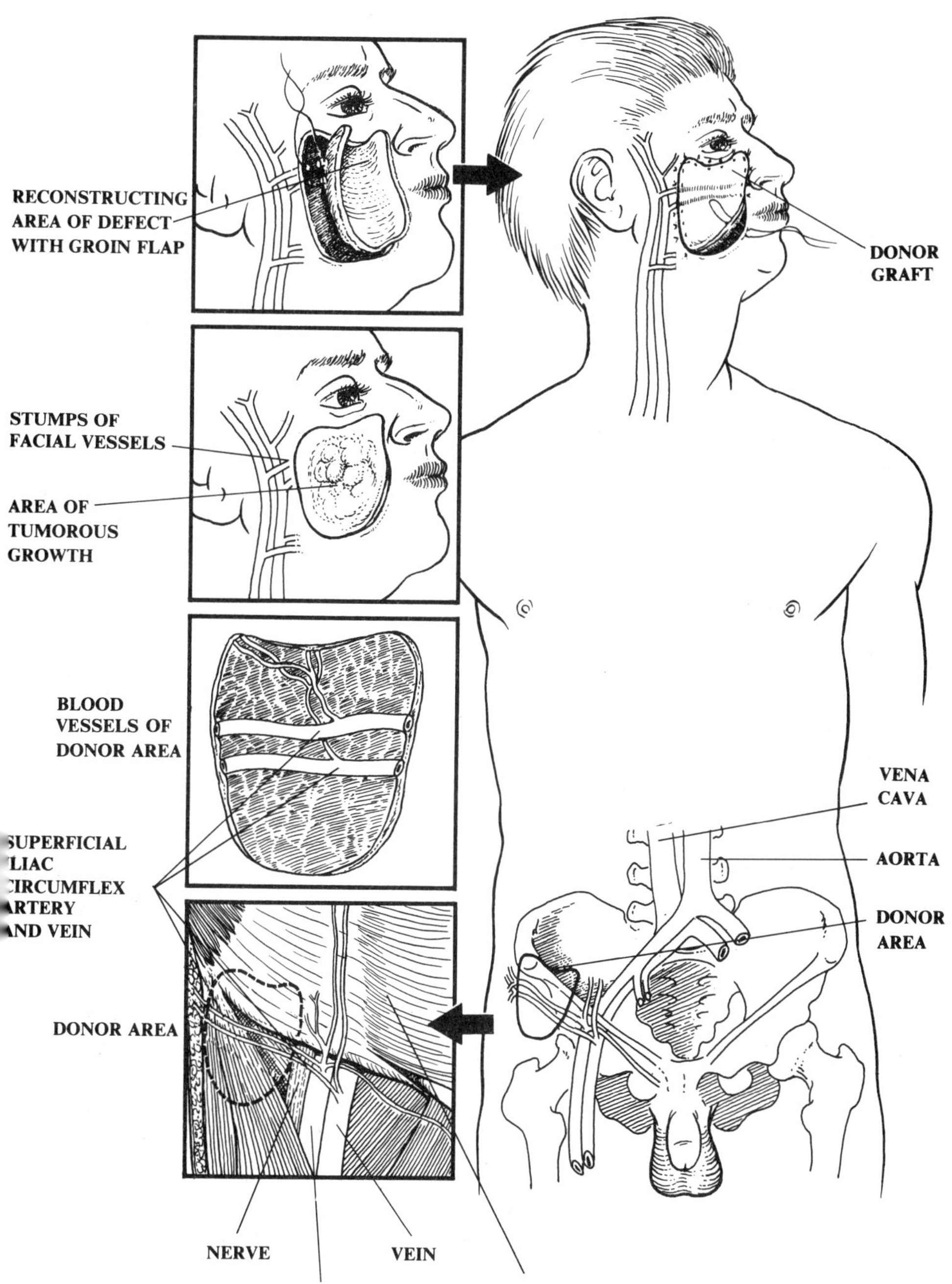

The Donor Graft

Diagram of transferring groin tissue to the face via microvascular surgery

Skin Tumors

Skin tumors, both benign and malignant, are easy to see and easy to treat in their early stages, easier by far than tumorous growths that occur in internal organs. Many skin lesions are so distinctive that a surgeon can usually tell at first sight whether or not they are malignant. If a surgeon is reasonably sure that a lesion is malignant he will have an excisional biopsy performed. When this is done the lesion is totally removed, and examined by a pathologist to confirm the diagnosis.

When a lesion is near the mouth, nose, eyelids, or other cosmetically important but difficult to reconstruct areas that may require surgical treatment, a definite pathological diagnosis is made before the lesion is completely removed. Only part of the growth will be removed for the incisional biopsy.

Your surgeon may elect to take a piece of a questionable lesion and have it examined pathologically before he decides whether or not to operate. A slight delay in performing the operation should not affect the prognosis.

A tumor, of course, does not have to be malignant; many are benign. A benign tumor has cells that behave in an orderly and predictable manner and do not invade surrounding tissues. Malignant tumors do invade and destroy.

Skin cancer is the most common type of malignancy; it also has the highest rate of cure. While the number of new cases discovered each year is about 100,000, annual deaths from skin cancer are only about 4,000. The incidence of skin cancer in the United States is higher in the South, and that's probably due to the sun. Because of this, people with skin cancer must avoid overexposure to the sun's rays. Sun "blockers" are effective; they include products containing a derivative of para-aminobenzoic acid that blocks out the ultraviolet rays of the sun. Sun "tanners" are not as effective a shield.

Carcinoma can develop anywhere on the skin, including the ear. Men who are outdoors a lot occasionally get a little growth on the ear; it is usually removed easily. Sometimes, however, the cartilage has to be taken out and the ear must be surgically reconstructed.

More men than women, about three to one, get skin cancer. That's probably because of outdoor work and resultant increased sun exposure. It is not a condition found in young men, as a rule. Few cases occur in men under forty; the majority are in their sixties and older.

X rays and chemicals also have been known to be causes for the increasing incidence of skin cancer. X rays for the removal of facial hair or correction of acne are now considered dangerous, frequently resulting in skin cancer many years down the road. The coal tar derivatives found in certain industrial oils have been discovered to be further causative agents in skin cancer development.

Skin cancers can also develop from burn scars. Such scars are notoriously unstable, particularly if they have been allowed to heal by themselves without a skin graft. If the scar is at a joint, such as the knee or elbow, where it is subject to constant flexion, the unstable scars have a greater chance of breaking down. When there are chronic areas of ulceration as a result of old burns, full thickness skin grafts should be utilized in order to prevent the chronic breakdown of the area and the potential development of subsequent skin cancer.

You should seek prompt medical attention when a skin growth appears and persists for four or five weeks without resolution. You may observe that the growth heals and then reoccurs, and that it is susceptible to bleeding when touched even slightly. The nonhealing ulcer that bleeds is one of the hallmarks of skin cancer.

Malignant tumors of the skin are primarily either basal- or squamous-cell (a more aggressive type of tumor) in origin, depending on the level of the skin in which they occur. Most skin tumors are basal cell in origin. The squamous cell is the more dangerous because it has the greater potential for spreading. Squamous-cell carcinoma can appear in any part of the body, but about 70 to 80 percent occur in the facial area. It can also occur on the hands.

The skin that contains squamous-cell carcinoma can be recognized as a raised, thickened area with a central crater or dimple, and with the surrounding skin frequently firm and elevated.

In a small percentage of cases there will be spreading to the lymph nodes or glands of the surrounding area. Your doctor therefore will routinely examine areas of potential lymph-node drainage surrounding the tumor. If the tumor occurs in the head or neck area, the doctor will examine the glands in the neck. If a lesion occurs on the back of the hand, the glands in the armpit, or axilla, will be examined.

Basal-cell carcinoma usually spreads at a much slower rate. The lesions are generally raised, have tiny blood vessels on the surface, and frequently bleed when touched. They do not usually spread to lymph nodes. Unless the condition is neglected for a very long time the prognosis for cure is excellent.

The key to cure with all of these tumors is complete removal. Special care and treatment is needed when the surgery is around the eyelids, mouth, or nose so as to avoid deformity. The best cosmetic result is achieved when there is early detection. Advanced cases frequently require multiple procedures.

Treatment varies. X-ray treatment, electrodesiccation and cautery, excision of the lesion, and closure by pulling the skin edges together or by applying skin grafts are all acceptable methods.

The method of treatment I prefer is excision and then closure, either by advancing the local skin or by applying a skin graft. The surgical removal of the lesion and the examination of it by a pathologist to make sure that all cancerous elements have been removed presents the best chance of cure. I do not care to burn or cauterize these lesions because I cannot be sure that all the malignant cells are destroyed. I *am* convinced when the pathologist reports to me: "Lesion is completely excised and all margins are free." I then have reasonable security that the lesion is adequately removed.

While smaller lesions can be adequately removed in an office complex, larger lesions should be removed in a hospital, where the surgeon can be sure, through pathology tests, that the entire tumor is eliminated. A plastic surgeon will not be afraid to cut away a little bit extra in order to assure himself fully that there is no further malignancy present. He knows that no matter how large an excision has to be made, he can reconstruct it by a variety of means. The reconstruction is usually done immediately following the excision.

Melanoma

Melanoma is a more serious malignancy and can arise in any cell of the body. Melanin, the pigmented substance within the deeper

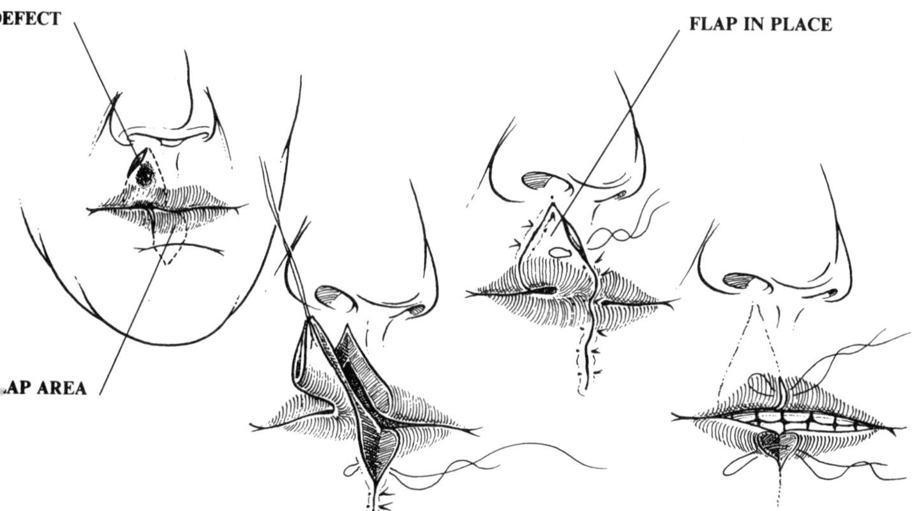

The Abbé Flap

The Abbé or cross-lip flap is the technique by which large tumors of either the upper or lower lip can be excised and reconstructed without severe distortion by utilizing smaller segments of the opposing lip.

layers of the skin, gives the skin its characteristic color. Not all lesions that are pigmented, however, are melanomas. The incidence of melanoma actually is quite low; the ratio is four in one hundred thousand as compared to, say, carcinoma in the colon, which occurs approximately in thirty cases out of every hundred thousand. Nonetheless, any pigmented lesion, particularly one that changes color, size, or shape, or one that ulcerates, bleeds, or itches should be checked out by a physician. If the physician thinks it is suspicious he probably will suggest that a surgeon remove it.

These tumors are usually excised widely, making it difficult to close the site of the excision. Skin grafting may therefore be required. As with all tumors, the best results occur after early diagnosis. Excision and a pathology examination will determine if further surgical procedures are necessary.

Leukoplakia

Leukoplakia is a condition in which white patches develop on the inside of the mouth and along the tongue. These elevated white patches can be caused by the sun, tobacco, poorly fitted dentures, or bad teeth. At one time it was felt that leukoplakia was a premalignant condition, but that belief is not widely held today. The lesions usually can be improved by taking away the offending agent; that is, by getting better fitting dentures or cutting out the use of tobacco. If the lesion persists, despite good oral hygiene, it is wise to have a biopsy performed.

Leukoplakic lesions can be treated surgically by removing the area and allowing it to heal by itself. The oral mucous membranes (tissue lining the mouth and tongue) have tremendous regenerative powers.

Freckles

Frequently, pigmented lesions usually found on the face and the hands appear early in life; they will darken during the summer and fade in the winter. They are more often seen in fair-haired, blue-eyed individuals.

There are many freckle haters who have gone to plastic surgeons to see about their removal. Some may claim that there are procedures that help—ones that involve the superficial destruction of the skin. Various acids, such as trichloracetic acid, are applied, as well as carbon dioxide slush and liquid nitrogen. Results vary, but from my experience, these treatments can result in unpredictable pigment changes in the skin. Freckles on the face, back of hand, or back are best left alone.

Port-Wine Stains

The port-wine stain, or purplish discoloration, is most observable when it is on the facial area, but it can also appear on the chest, the scalp, and down the neck. The disfigurement is caused by an enlargement of the capillaries, or blood vessels, in the dermal, or deeper, layer of the skin. At present there is no corrective procedure that provides entirely satisfactory results. In the past, men had the area tattooed to cover up the stains. Makeup has also been applied as a temporary and not very acceptable solution. The removal of the area and its replacement by a skin graft also gives results that are not always acceptable.

The most promising answer to the problem may lie in laser-beam technology. A few medical centers are experimenting in this area.

Strawberry Marks

Strawberry marks, or capillary-type tumors, are bright red or bluish soft lesions that are elevated above the surrounding skin. They usually appear a few months after birth and reach maximum size when the child is about one year old. While quite disturbing to the family at the time, the marks generally disappear by the time the child starts school, at about age five.

You can tell that the strawberry mark is becoming resolved by the appearance of the so-called "herald patch"—a grayish area that indicates that the blood vessels are involuting and scarring down. The patch may ultimately leave some scarring, but it generally is negligible compared to the original condition.

So, when a strawberry mark appears on an infant, the best treatment is first to watch and wait. In most instances the mark will disappear and leave only a slightly scarred residual area. But if the mark begins to grow and ulcerate—and particularly if it occurs about the mouth area—surgical excision may be necessary. Excision frequently requires reconstruction of the area around the mouth at a later date.

There is another kind of blood vessel tumor, but, unlike the strawberry mark, it is located in the deeper, softer tissues—most often in the head and neck area. Called cavernous hemangioma, it is characterized by sacs, or spaces, that are filled with blood in the loose tissues of the body below the skin. If they expand and enlarge to a marked degree, surgery may be required.

Cleft Lip and Cleft Palate

What is technically known as a cleft lip is known to the layman public as a "harelip." The cleft palate and lip are embryological defects caused by a failure of the tissues of the left and right side of the face to grow together. The incidence of cleft lips is about one in 1,400 live births.

There are different types of palate clefts: unilateral clefts, bilateral clefts, and clefts of the lip. There can also be clefts farther back on the hard palate—all the way to the back of the throat—as well as isolated clefts of the hard palate and isolated clefts of the soft palate.

In treating such conditions, surgical techniques involve closure of the cleft lip and palate with fine suture material under a minimum of tension. The results are usually quite rewarding.

The treatment of a youngster with a cleft lip and palate requires a multidisciplinary approach. The orthodontist, prosthodontist, and plastic surgeon, together with the ear, nose, and throat surgeon, are all part of the reconstruction team.

The patient can have more than cosmetic problems. A hearing loss may develop: when the palate is open the ears are susceptible to infection as the middle-ear canal drains back into the throat. There can also be regurgitation of food through the nose and there can be difficulty in breathing. Where the palate is too short and doesn't close off the nasal area, a child will have nasal speech and will require speech therapy.

The usual surgical plan calls for closure of the cleft lip at about twelve weeks of age. It is performed by a plastic surgeon while the child is under general anesthesia. The palate is operated on when the child is about one year old.

The soft palate is closed early in the child's life because speech patterns are ingrained early, and it is felt that the sooner the palatal split is put together, the better the child's speech pattern can be.

FIFTEEN

The Hand

BESIDES being an essential appendage used to grasp and hold objects, the hand is also important to us creatively and psychologically. Almost as much can be discerned from watching the movements of a man's hands as from noticing the expression on his face. In fact, the hand is second only to the face in portraying the human personality. Nervousness, anger, warmth, hostility—all these emotions are communicated with the hands. And often it is fairly easy to estimate an individual's age accurately by studying his hands.

Physiology of the Hand

What is this highly complex part of the anatomy called the hand? First, it is composed of skin, underlying firmer tissue, or fascia, and subcutaneous tissue containing fat. Then there are the bones and joints, muscles, tendons, nerves, and blood vessels. All of these intricate structures play a part in the hand's overall functioning, and traumatic injuries can occur to any or all of the structures. The seriousness of such injuries often depends on the number of structures that are involved.

The skin firmly adheres to the palm of the hand, while it is much looser on the hand's top surface; try pinching your skin at the top of the hand versus the palm to see the difference. The main function of the skin is to protect the underlying structures. A serious wound of the skin can cause malfunctioning of the hand; for example, an injury that results in contractures and scarring can prevent normal functioning and movement of the fingers. The skin of the hand is also subject to a multiplicity of tumors that may require treatment.

The framework of the hand is composed of three sets of bones: the carpal bones of the wrist, the five metacarpal bones of the palm, and

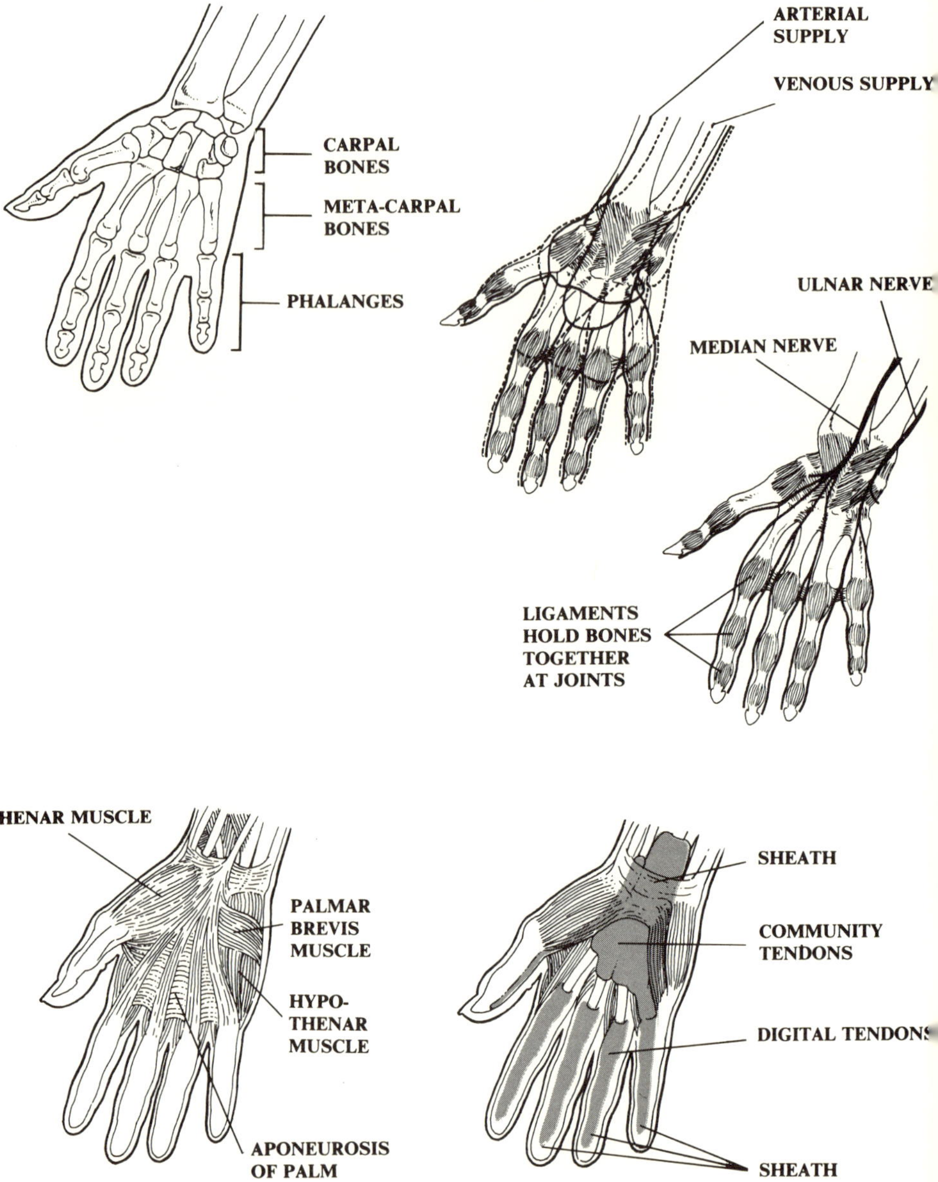

CARPAL BONES
META-CARPAL BONES
PHALANGES

ARTERIAL SUPPLY
VENOUS SUPPLY

ULNAR NERVE
MEDIAN NERVE
LIGAMENTS HOLD BONES TOGETHER AT JOINTS

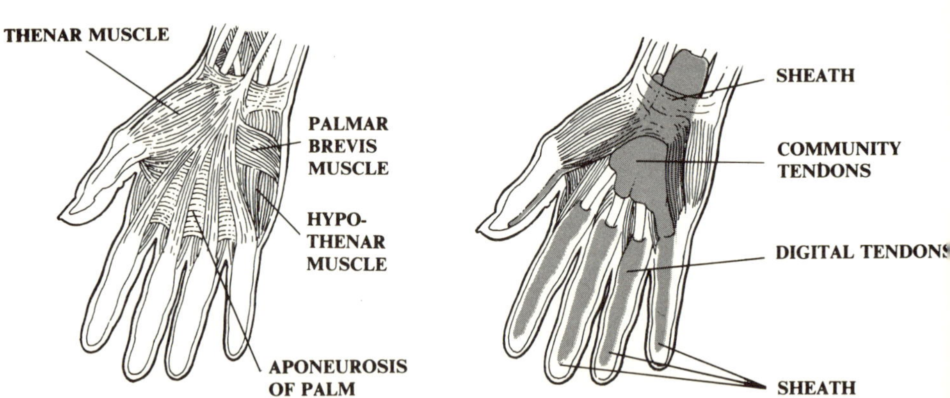

The Anatomy of the Hand

A. The basic bony framework of the hand. Twenty-eight bones comprise the fingers, hand, and wrist.

B. The blood supply of the hand showing the intricate network of arteries and veins.

C. The major nerve supply of the hand. These nerves provide sensation and the impulse to move the muscles.

D. The superficial muscles

E. The tendons and their covering.

the phalanges—the bones that make up the digits. In order to interact with each other, these bones are connected by joints and ligaments. Injury to one set of bones can have direct influence upon the other contiguous set of bones.

Muscles and tendons are responsible for the movements of the digits. They, in turn, function because of the nerves in the hand. Damage to the nerves can result in loss of sensation and ultimately in severe injury to the hand because of the loss of protective sensation that the nerves provide. Similarly, the loss of motor nerves supplying the electric stimulus to the muscles of the hand results in its inability to function.

Surgery of the hand is highly specialized and, though a plastic surgeon must have a detailed knowledge of its anatomy, those who do essentially cosmetic work may refer such operations to a specialist, e.g., an orthopedic surgeon with a specialty in surgery of the hand or to a plastic surgeon who is doing the surgery on a regular basis.

The Reasons for Surgery

The natural effects of the aging process leave their marks on the hand. Often a man's face will look young, but his hands will betray his true age. These age marks—spots and darkened freckles, wrinkled skin, excessive folds—appear on most men's hands eventually, but little in the way of cosmetic correction can be done. Surgery is available to restore the function of the hand, and to correct its deformities, but in most situations the cosmetic wonders we can perform on the face and body do not work as well on the hand.

Like other parts of the body, the hand is also subject to certain diseases: from benign cysts to the development of tumorous growths of skin, tendon, bone, muscle, and nerve, not to mention arthritic conditions. There are also traumatic injuries to the hand, as well as congenital situations in which children are born with missing, malpositioned, or extra fingers, and congenital abnormalities of the upper extremities. Surgical correction of these disorders is also within the province of the surgeon whose specialty is the hand.

• • •

CONDITIONS OF THE HAND AND SURGICAL PROCEDURES

The surgical procedure performed always depends on the part of the hand that is affected and the type of injury that is sustained. Following are brief descriptions of those areas of the hand most frequently injured and the surgical procedure that is employed.

The Nail

The nail is a complex structure with some of the characteristics of the hair. Composed of a growing part, the cuticle area, which contains the general matrix from which the nail grows—about one millimeter per week in the fingers, and only about half that rate in the toes—a complete fingernail will grow out in approximately four to five months.

A physician can tell a great deal about you from an examination of your nails. They may indicate certain diseases and processes that might be present in your system. Blood conditions can be detected through the nail bed—a pale nail can indicate anemia, while a darkly reddened nail may show evidence of congenital heart disease. The so-called cherry-red color of the nail bed may be caused by carbon monoxide poisoning. Scalings that are taken of the nail for fungal analysis will often determine the cause of disturbed or retarded growth, and the offending organism can be treated. The degree of hardness and the brittle quality of your nails can also indicate the state of your nutrition and whether or not your diet can be considered adequate.

Nails are also subject to tumors. The so-called glomus tumors are blood-vessel types that cause extreme tenderness and pain over the nail bed; certain tumors may even be malignant although the incidence is rare.

Nail growth can be slowed down or disturbed by disease, malnutrition, and/or acute illnesses. When this occurs you may frequently notice grooves across the nail, representing the different growth patterns that indicate periods of normal health by smoothness and illness by ridges. Transverse bands can occur as the result of various poisonings; arsenic, for instance, produces a white band across the nail.

Many injuries that result in a crushed nail distort the growing plane of the nail and will ultimately disturb the nail's growth and appearance. An accident that crushes the nail may cause an accumulation of blood beneath it. This extremely painful condition is treated by a physician by passing a small needle or pin through the nail bed so that the blood is released; once the blood is allowed to pass through, the pain resolves itself.

A relatively common wound of the finger itself involves the loss of the soft tissues from its top or side. This may be caused by an accident from a knife, tool, or piece of machinery. The result can be exposure of tendons, muscles, and bone, and may require soft-tissue coverage from adjacent areas. Less severe injuries that do not expose deeper structures merely require a split-thickness piece of skin (usually 10 to 13 millimeters). It is important to bear in mind that prompt surgical attention to any injury involving loss of tissue will usually give a better result and help minimize long-term disability.

The Tendon

The tendon is the prime mover of the fingers. Along with the surrounding bones, nerves, and soft tissue, it is frequently involved in any injury. Since all of these structures are close to each other and have different healing potentials, and because one structure can fuse with another, quick medical attention to repair the injured area is advisable.

The tendon lies in a tubelike structure composed of fibrous and bony tissue with a surrounding lubricating fluid; it glides smoothly within the tube. When injured, the tendon and tube will frequently adhere to each other, so that there can be postoperative limitations of hand movement and the gliding motion can be lost. Early mobility and physical therapy (within three to four weeks after surgery) can decrease the possibility of tendon adherence to the surrounding tissue, and allow for better functioning following any injury.

Nerves

Nerves are similar to the multiple strands in telephone cables. While some nerves have sensory functions, others give electric impulses to move muscles. There are hundreds of strands in a single nerve. Each strand has a precise purpose; all the strands working together allow for smooth functioning of the hand.

Injury to the nerves presents a complex problem to the surgeon. If the nerves are severed they cannot be individually reunited even under the best of microsurgical techniques. The most that can be hoped for is to get the severed ends to meet as closely as possible, so that protective sensation can be restored in the area of the skin. Great strides, however, have been made lately in microvascular surgery. Microscopic magnification enables surgeons to work more effectively with minute nerve ends, allowing better approximation and helping to restore some of the lost functions.

Pain and numbness of the hand, particularly at night, are common symptoms of a specific condition. This situation results when one or two of the major nerves of the hand are trapped or compressed in a narrow tunnel surrounded by the unyielding bony structures and tendons of the wrist. Symptoms frequently occur during sleep when an individual inadvertently flexes the wrist, which further compresses the nerves. Splinting of the wrist and an occasional injection of steroids into the area may help in certain cases. However, if the condition persists and there is a muscular weakness or loss of substance to the muscle, surgery may be indicated. (A diagnostic test frequently performed prior to surgery involves measuring the conduction or transmission of the nerve current to determine if there is any latency or blockage.)

If surgery is indicated, the procedure involves incisions over the areas where the nerves are entrapped. Surgical techniques can free the nerve. After the operation a splint is applied, and remains for several weeks, so that the area can heal while immobilized.

Bones

Fractures of the bones of the hand can be treated by surgical procedures, or by the application of a splint or cast to immobilize the fractured parts. Either procedure is aimed at good healing and arranging of the small fracture fragments in a good position. Depending on the location of the fracture, immobility is recommended from periods of two to six weeks.

Fractures near or through the joints or bony articulations are more apt to lead to limitations of the involved joint. That is why, as in all hand injuries, prompt attention may minimize post-traumatic disability.

Ganglia

A ganglion is a nodular-like growth, frequently occurring in the wrist area, either on the palmar surface or on the top of the wrist near the thumb/wrist articulation, and is often related to stress in the area in which it occurs. The ganglion cyst, usually filled with gelatinous material, grows slowly and elevates the skin above it. Generally there is a stalk that reaches to the tendon and bone underneath. This benign growth can be a severe annoyance, but it is routinely treated with good results.

One antiquated method of rupturing a ganglion was done with a heavy book, but really the best way to remove one is to aspirate it with a needle, or to operate on the area. Removal with a large needle generally is worth the effort, because when successful it avoids surgery. My own experience, however, has been that ganglia must usually be removed through a surgical procedure. An overnight stay in a hospital would be required for removal of the cyst. A splint would also be applied for a week or so in order to immobilize the area during healing.

Warts

The common wart, or *verruca vulgaris,* is caused by a virus. Treatment varies greatly here; everything—including suggestive psychotherapy, coagulation, application of strong acids, coring out the lesions, cryo (cold knife) surgery—has been tried with different results. Most procedures will produce some improvement of these lesions; in fact, with time they usually resolve themselves. But still a growth of warts can be a persistent annoyance.

Surgical excision can be more trouble than the unsightly nature of a wart is worth, particularly when the skin defects caused by the lesions have to be closed. The reason: closure of the skin is a problem because warts frequently occur over areas of the palm of the hand and the tops of the fingers, where there is not an abundance of skin.

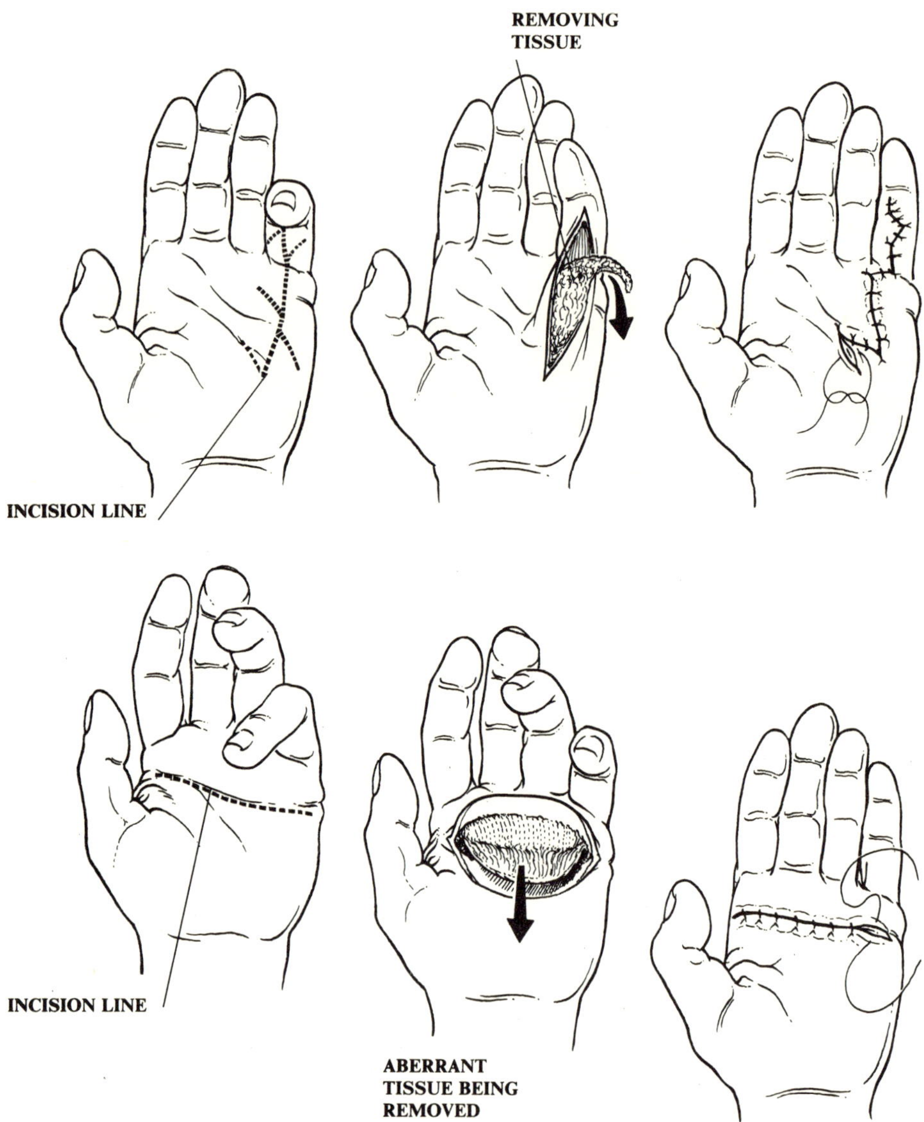

Hand Surgery for Correction of Dupuytren's Contracture

A. The zig-zag incision on the finger. This zig-zag is used to avoid contracture of the skin upon healing.

B. The fibrous tissue being removed.

C. The incisions have been closed with "darts" at the finger and hand creases to avoid any contractures while healing.

D. The incision used to remove the fibrous tissue in the palm, another common area for Dupuytren's contracture.

E. The removal of the dense fibrous tissue from the palm.

F. Closure of the transverse incision.

Tumors

Tumors, either benign or malignant, can develop in any part of the hand. A surgeon will frequently perform an excisional biopsy or a partial removal of the lesion, which is sent to a laboratory for pathology examination. If the tumor is benign, a less extensive excision is possible than if the lesion were malignant.

I might add that many seemingly unimportant lesions of the hand are unfortunately allowed to remain undiagnosed for too long. If they are malignant, removal at an earlier stage can provide greater assurance of a cure.

The Palm

A thickening of the tissues of the palm is known as Dupuytren's contracture. A hereditary basis has also been established for this condition; it is more common among Celtic people, and almost never occurs among blacks or Asians. It may be but is not necessarily related to an occupational trauma and when severe is best treated by surgery so that the offending scar tissue can be removed. Other diseases of the palm can vary from a small nodule in the palm of the hand to a more extensive thickening fibrosis of the palm tissues. Where large painful nodules interfere with function, or where contracting tissue pulls down the fourth and fifth fingers into the palm, surgery is usually recommended. The procedure here involves incisions in the palm and removal of scar tissue. Occasionally skin grafting and rotation of local skin flaps are also necessary to cover or replace the skin that has been destroyed by the underlying scar tissue. Dupuytren's contracture is a benign process that can end up being quite disabling. It can be treated successfully in most cases.

Fingers

Extra digits, webbed fingers, and other rare congenital birth abnormalities are usually corrected before the patient is of school age. Severe congenital problems of the hand may require multiple procedures.

Glossary

abdominal lipectomy: The procedure for removal of excess abdominal skin and fat.

anti-helix: The folded portion of the ear, frequently missing in congenital ear deformities—the so-called "lop" ear.

benign: Refers to a lesion that is not malignant.

blepharoplasty: The term for cosmetic surgery of the eyelids. Derived from the Greek *blepharos,* eye.

cartilage: The supporting framework of the ear, nose, etc.

cephalometrics: The study of the relationship of the facial parts to each other; used in facial reconstruction.

chemical peeling: The application of phenol to the skin to soften fine lines and wrinkles.

chemosurgery: The application of chemicals to the skin to remove lesions and pigmented areas, and to firm up the skin, as in chemical peeling.

coagulation process: The protein components of the skin are denatured by chemicals such as phenol or TCA. Upon skin regeneration, a smooth appearance occurs.

collagen: A major structural component of the skin. It is a molecule and consists of a three-coil polypeptide chain made of amino acids (protein).

dermabrasion: The process by which the upper layer of skin is removed; commonly used for post-acne scars.

dermal: Referring to the second layer of skin, which contains hair follicles and sweat glands.

dermoplaning: The process by which the upper layer of the skin is surgically removed by means of a hand-held planing apparatus.

ectropion: The pulling away of the lower lid, occasionally seen following lower-lid surgery; usually temporary and treated by taping the lower lid for a short period of time.

elastic fibers: Protein fibers that give support to the dermal layer of the skin.

epidermis: The upper layer of the skin that is constantly being replaced by the deeper dermal layer.

epispadias: A condition in which the urethra opens up at the top of the penis, rather than the end.

general anesthesia: Administration of a drug to render the patient unconscious, and during which no pain sensation is present under surgery.

gynecomastia: Excessive development of the male mammary glands. A common, temporary occurrence in normal adolescence, it usually resolves itself by age twenty-one.

hair follicles: The bulblike structures from which the hair shafts grow.

helix: The folded rim of cartilage forming the margin of the ear.

hematoma: A collection of blood beneath the skin following surgery. It occurs infrequently. Prompt detection and removal prevent any serious complications.

hypertrophic scar: An elevated scar that usually flattens with time.

hypospadias: A developmental anomaly in which the urethra (urinary canal) opens on the undersurface of the penis rather than the end.

keloid: A benign abnormal growth of scar tissue occasionally following a skin incision. May be resistant to treatment.

local anesthesia: Opposed to general; the operative site is sufficiently numbed to allow surgery without requiring the patient to be totally unconscious.

malignant: Refers to a growth that has an uncontrollable pattern and may spread. Surgery in the early stage offers the best cure.

mandible: The lower jaw.

melanin: Pigmented granules found in the deeper layer of the skin. They are responsible for the skin's coloration.

mentoplasty: A procedure to change the structure of the chin. Usually means chin augmentation via silicone implant.

microtia: The condition of absence of the external ear.

microvascular surgery: The surgery of small blood vessels and nerves. An increasingly used procedure for digital and limb re-implantation.

novocaine: (Xylocaine). The local anesthetic most commonly used for plastic surgery.

osteotomy: The cutting of bone anywhere in the body, usually for the purpose of repositioning it.

otoplasty: The technical term for correction of external-ear abnormalities, variations, or deformities.

phenol: The chemical most commonly used for face-peeling procedures.

plugs: Devices used in the hair transplantation procedure. The round 4- to 5-mm. plug contains scalp and ten to fifteen hairs within its follicles.

prognathism: A prominent lower-jaw condition.

ptosis: A falling or sinking-down of an organ or structure.

rhinoplasty: From the Greek word *rhinos,* nose, and the technical term for nasal surgery.

rhytidectomy: A face-lift.

scalp flap: The rotation of hair-bearing skin from the sides and the back of the scalp to the front.

Silastic: Trade name used for the siliconized rubber used in surgery.

silicone: A plastic based on silicon. It can be safely implanted in the human without rejection.

skin planing: The removal of the upper layers of skin. Another term for dermabrasion.

steroids: A family of chemical substances comprising many hormones and vitamins. Some steroids can be injected into scars to soften them.

strip graft: A long and narrow segment of hair-bearing scalp, taken from the back of the scalp and placed in the front of the scalp to construct an anterior hairline.

TCA: Trichloracetic acid. One of the chemicals used to remove superficial skin lesions and discolorations.

undereye bags: A lay term to describe prominent bulging of the lower-lid area due to a pushing-out of excess fat that surrounds the eye.

Index

Numbers in italics indicate illustrations